HOW TO CHOOSE A NURSING HOME

HOW TO CHOOSE A NURSING HOME

A Guide To Quality Caring

JOANNE MESHINSKY, R.N.

AVON BOOKS ⬥ NEW YORK

This book is offered to the memory of my parents,
Anna and Joseph Pluto

HOW TO CHOOSE A NURSING HOME: A GUIDE TO QUALITY CARING is an original publication of Avon Books. This work has never before appeared in book form.

AVON BOOKS
A division of
The Hearst Corporation
105 Madison Avenue
New York, New York   10016

Copyright © 1991 by Joanne Meshinsky
Published by arrangement with the author
Library of Congress Catalog Card Number: 90-45289
ISBN: 0-380-76078-9

Library of Congress Cataloging in Publication Data:
Meshinsky, Joanne E.
  How to choose a nursing home : a guide to quality caring / Joanne E. Meshinsky.
  p. cm.
  Includes bibliographical references and index.
  1. Nursing homes—Evaluation. 2. Nursing home care—Evaluation.
3. Consumer education. I. Title.
RA997.M47   1991
362.1′6—dc20   90-45289

First Avon Books Trade Printing: February 1991

AVON TRADEMARK REG. U.S. PAT. OFF. AND IN OTHER COUNTRIES, MARCA REGISTRADA.
HECHO EN U.S.A.

Printed in the U.S.A.

OPM 10 9 8 7 6 5 4 3 2 1

Contents

Preface and Acknowledgments   vii

Introduction   1
  Quality of Life   1
  The Decision to Look for a Nursing Home   5
  Using This Book   10

1. How Nursing Homes Are Regulated   15
  How Nursing Homes Are Classified   15
    Personal Care Nursing Homes   16
    Intermediate Care Nursing Homes   17
    Skilled Care Nursing Homes   17
    Multilevel Nursing Homes   17
    Chronic Care Facilities   17
  What Inspectors Look For   19
  Public Reports and How to Get Them   25
  Substandard Nursing Homes   26

2. How Nursing Homes Operate   30
  Administrator   31
  Medical Director   33
  Director of Nurses   34
  Clinical Nurse Manager (Charge or Head Nurse)   36
  Certified Medicine Aide   37
  Geriatric Nursing Assistant   38
  Social Worker   39
  Activities Director   40
  Therapists   42
  Dietitian   43
  Housekeeping, Laundry, and Maintenance Workers   45
  The Interdisciplinary Patient Care Plan   46

3. Choosing a Nursing Home   48
  Seeking Referrals   49
  Touring the Facility   50
  Talking to Residents and Staff   53
  Evaluating Care   55
  Comparing Nursing Homes   60

4. **Arranging for Payments**   **63**
   Using Private Sources   65
   Medicare   67
     Part A   68
     Part B   71
   Medicaid   72
   Fraudulent Charges   75

5. **Moving to a Nursing Home**   **78**
   Feelings about the Change   78
   Preparations   80
   Paperwork   83
   What to Bring, What to Leave at Home   84
   The First Day   87
   Adjustments   89

6. **Living in a Nursing Home**   **94**
   Everyday Medical Problems   94
   Disease and Disability   98
   Pain Control   103
   Supplemental Medical Services   105
   The Resident and the Family   107
   Discharge   109

7. **Handling Problems**   **112**
   Abuse and Inadequate Care   113
   Problems with Staff Members   117
   Questions about the Doctor   120
   What to Do   121

8. **Dying in a Nursing Home**   **125**
   AIDS   126
   The Stages of Dying   128
   When Death Occurs   133

Afterword: Working for Change   **135**
   Government Action   135
   Citizen Involvement   136

Appendix A. A Resident's Bill of Rights   **138**
                 Example of Complaint Procedure   140
Appendix B. Directory of State Agencies on Aging   **141**
Appendix C. Directory of Health Facility Licensing and
                 Certification Directors   149
Appendix D. Resource Centers for the Needs and
                 Concerns of the Elderly   **160**
Appendix E. Drugs in Geriatrics   **164**

Glossary of Medical Terms   **168**

Bibliography   **175**

Index   **179**

Preface and Acknowledgments

This book began with my son's suggestion that I write a newspaper column on nursing homes based on my experience. I have been a geriatric nurse in long-term care facilities for over fifteen years and have also been the relative of a nursing home resident; my father spent a period of time during his terminal illness in a nursing home. After considering my son's suggestion and my own belief that the public needs accurate information about the "inner workings" of nursing homes, I decided to write this book, to give the insider's view of nursing homes and to offer help and practical guidance to those searching for appropriate placement for a loved one.

Recent events have focused public attention on nursing homes. The Institute of Medicine Committee on Nursing Home Regulations embarked on a study that ultimately changed the inspection rules of nursing homes, thereby strengthening resident rights and quality of care. The country's awareness of the aging population has been expanded by the magnificent job done by Senator John Heinz (R-Pa.), who chaired the Senate Special Committee on Aging, and by Representative Claude Pepper (D-Fla.), who spent his life beating the drum in support of our "old-old" citizens. Now Senator David Pryor (D-Ark.) has taken over and is striving to improve the quality of care to the elderly, with Senators John Melcher (D-Mont.) and George Mitchell (D-Maine) proposing their own agendas on behalf of the aging. From Hollywood, actor Kirk Douglas has brought his considerable prestige to bear on the problems facing the elderly. Such public support shows a welcome recognition of the elderly's problems.

This book is designed to complement such public support by offering personal experience and practical information to the elderly and their families. My book will tell you about the negative as well as the positive aspects of nursing home living because I believe you need and deserve to know all sides of the issue of geriatric care. Placing a loved one in a long-term care facility is an awesome responsibility, one often fraught with painful emotions: doubt, apprehension, and guilt. *How to Choose a Nursing Home: A Guide to Quality Caring* offers help, advice, and encouragement to make the task less difficult.

To all who have provided substance for this book—nursing home personnel, friends, relatives, the residents and their families—I give my heartfelt thanks. Whatever benefit derives from this effort is the result of your support and encouragement.

Personal thanks are due many people and organizations for the numerous hours they devoted to my cause in the midst of their own. In the initial stages, Kathleen Phillips supported my endeavors and edited the first draft of the manuscript; Steve Krauss researched and typed; and Betty Mawby, a former director of nurses in geriatrics, provided insights into care planning. Dr. Thomas Ward, a medical director of a long-term care facility, volunteered to read the manuscript and made helpful suggestions by contributing his vast knowledge of nursing home policies. Dave Houston, pharmacist, supplied current drug information and read the section on drug usage in the elderly. Dr. Steve Lipson, director of a long-term care facility, then added his expertise and help on drugs used in the elderly and on the book's glossary of medical terms. Beverly Krueger, R.N., supplied additional information on nursing home surveyors' observations. Norma Fraley, R.N., D.O.N., provided input on skilled rehabilitation services. Joan Lubitz, R.N., collected numerous resource materials and names of organizations that help the elderly and their families. Helen McNesby, R.N., former co-worker, helped to refresh my memory on past events and then added her suggestions and additions for the book after a member of her own family was admitted to a nursing home.

When she heard of the project, Joanne Livingston, R.N.C., B.S., rescued me from the hours of research needed to update portions of the book by reviewing my comments on the many aspects of quality of life in long-term care facilities and providing dates of implementation of new federal regulations. Joanne continues in her daily efforts and commitment toward ensuring excellence in long-term care.

I am grateful to Linda Clark, executive vice-president of

Delmarva Foundation for Medical Care, for her continual support to all involved in long-term and acute care. It's been said that "when you want something done right give it to a busy person," and so I gave my manuscript to Linda to help in the updating of regulatory information. Carla Murray, R.N., also shared her expertise in the Medicare regulations.

Karen Byrne-Hamilton, M.A./C.C.C.-S.L.P., took time from her busy schedule to explain a speech therapist's responsibilities.

Thanks are due to Ms. Nottingham, for supplying updated Licensure and Certification directories and to Allen Friedlob, for providing current nursing home statistics. I am indebted to Betty Cornelius, not only for the time and interest she gave me, but also for her help in bringing nursing home data and statistics into perspective.

With a sympathetic ear, support, energy, and years of editing expertise, Scott Chase and his wife, Lynn, came to my aid to contribute their professional help.

Many stages of the book benefited from Janet Gallant's excellent writing and editing skills and her unwavering belief in the need for more information on the subject of nursing homes. She not only contributed her knowledge but also volunteered her services to local nursing homes to assist in the high standard of care she believes our nation's elderly should receive.

I am grateful to my neighbor, Linda Aber, who directed me to Eileen Fallon, the most pleasant and diligent literary agent a first-time author could hope for.

And, finally, I am indebted to my editor at Avon Books, Judith Riven, for the suggestions and thought-provoking questions that helped me revise and thereby refine crucial topics throughout the book.

Not enough can be said to thank the many advocacy groups that keep families and caregivers alert to the needs and wants of the residents in nursing homes. To the long-term care surveyors and ombudsmen who daily are faced with decisions influencing policies on the quality of life in long-term care facilities, we offer our gratitude.

Special thanks are due my children—Jeff, Janine, and Michele—whose unstinting patience, good judgment, and gentle criticism kept me on course.

Most of all I want to thank John, my husband, who was

beside me night and day with words of encouragement, undaunting loyalty, and commitment to the topic of long-term care and who kept his sanity and serenity while teaching me to use the word processor.

Introduction

Quality of Life

This book is unlike any other you will read on finding a nursing home because it focuses on one of the most important issues of long-term care: the quality of life.

You are not alone if you are afraid of nursing homes—many people are. I often hear, "Nursing homes are depressing." "The people sit around all day with nothing to do." "Everyone's in a wheelchair, lined up against the walls." "It's a place to die." Many people refuse to talk about nursing homes, and some can't bring themselves to think about them, even when they or their family members are in need of one. What causes people to react in such a negative way? It is the widespread belief that entering a nursing home causes a drastic, irreversible decline in the quality of life—that a nursing home signals the end.

You will find, as you read this book, that a nursing home doesn't have to be a place of hopelessness, offering nothing to enhance a resident's life. I have spent my career as a geriatric nurse and I know that the quality of a person's life doesn't have to decline with admission to a good home. In fact, the quality of life can improve dramatically when people unable to care for themselves find encouragement and companionship in a nursing home that provides excellent care and values and protects its residents' rights.

Unfortunately, there are substandard homes. Newspaper articles, magazines, movies, and even your own neighbors' and relatives' stories testify to the existence of nursing homes where residents are exploited and abused, where even a simple request like "Please take me to the bathroom" may be met with indignation and insult.

You will have to search to find high-quality care. What might be keeping you from starting that search is fear—a fear based on stereotypes about nursing homes. Let's examine some of those stereotypes.

First, many people believe nursing homes are depressing, yet anyone who has spent time in nursing homes knows that often this is not the case. I have had wonderful and memorable times with residents. Through quiet conversations and listening, I have learned much about their lives and experiences, their travels, and their families. At other times residents have offered me valuable advice. I have been immeasurably enriched by their wisdom and knowledge, and their sense of humor has often lightened my heart. I clearly remember the day one nursing home resident smilingly said to me, "Age is a matter of mind: If you don't mind, it won't matter." I was taken aback by what she said, and I responded, "Mrs. M., you are so full of quips." She quickly turned to me with a puzzled look and answered, "That's funny, I don't remember eating any."

Another stereotype about nursing homes is that they are only for the elderly and the confused. In fact, many facilities are no longer devoted solely to the care of the elderly. Instead, the modern nursing home is for the recovery and recuperation of people of all ages. Even though the median age of residents in nursing homes is eighty-two, there are also those who are younger and infirm, those, for example, who have survived a car accident or drug overdose, or who are victims of debilitating diseases such as multiple sclerosis or AIDS. Many of those admitted to a nursing home may be there for less than ninety days. There are those who will remain only long enough to recover from a heart attack, broken bones, or surgery before returning home.

Many people believe in the stereotypical view of the nursing home as purely a medical facility: pills are given out and dressings are changed, but no attention is paid to the nonphysical needs of the residents. This, however, is not the case. Until the 1960s, nursing homes were scrutinized by the government and the public only for the physical aspects of care. As time went by, more components were added to assess the residents' quality of life. The focus broadened from merely physical issues to social, spiritual, and recreational ones. It became apparent to involved consumers, community activists, and concerned nursing home owners that all these aspects contribute to the quality of a resident's life. In the 1980s, an era of quality-of-life issues, it is no longer enough to look solely at the physical well-being of a nursing home resident. All nursing homes are required to identify a resident's physical, emotional, and spiritual needs and provide a plan of care to meet these needs. Only a facility that fulfills this obligation consistently will be known for the high quality of life it offers.

You may be wondering, "What *is* 'quality of life,' and is it really so important when all I want is a place for Mother to get nursing care?" Yes, quality of life is important, although different people may define it in different ways. Whatever makes you feel a high sense of self-esteem, dignity, self-assurance, security, emotional well-being, and physical comfort contributes to the quality of your life. Take these positive feelings away and you will be left with a devastating sense of loss and feeling of discomfort and displeasure. You may actually feel physically ill.

"Can quality of life be measured?" The answer is a qualified yes. As suggested by the Institute of Medicine (IoM), quality of life is measured by a process called "outcomes." Outcomes can be described as the result of care that has caused a change in a resident's functional or psychosocial behavior. Certainly there are some elements of care which are easier to identify than others. For instance, evaluators can easily judge the physical structures of a nursing home, but it is not so easy to measure residents' privacy needs and sexual needs.

One of the most important elements contributing to the quality of life is the degree to which a nursing home lets residents make choices. In the above-average facility, everything is done to ensure that residents will have choices in all aspects of care. For example, if a resident is used to going to bed at midnight, he should be allowed to stay awake until then if he so desires. Yet in some nursing homes, the residents will tell you they must prepare for bed immediately after dinner and that no one has a choice.

It may come as a surprise to you that in the best nursing homes, residents do a great deal for themselves. One of the indicators of a high quality of life is self-care, which does more to promote feelings of self-worth than having all of one's daily activities taken care of by someone else. Remember, most elderly people are used to taking care of themselves and others and feel very helpless having someone else wait on them. When you tour nursing homes you may even see residents making their own beds or dusting and cleaning out closets.

The best way to determine a nursing home's quality of life is to talk to the residents. Residents of above-average facilities are happy to share their experiences with you. And you can tell much by the conversations and behavior of residents in inferior homes. In the best of all possible worlds, if you needed a nursing home, you would find one that provided excellent care, was convenient, met all of your needs, and was affordable. However, it is rarely possible to find that ideal. The Senate Special Committee on Aging has said that finding high-quality patient care is a major problem and that the consumer has little control over the process. Since the beginning of Medicare's prospective payment system (PPS) and its financial incentives for hospitals to discharge patients earlier, some families have had to find nursing homes in a hurry. There are many excellent nursing homes from which to choose, but there are also some that do not place any emphasis on a resident's quality of life. You will have to seek out good care if you want the best living arrangement for your loved one, and it takes time to do this properly. The only way to prepare is to educate yourself.

While there are pamphlets and periodicals on nursing homes you can leaf through, you may still be in the dark about what goes on behind closed doors. General-information sources do not provide a picture of the entire nursing home scene. Such frequently heard advice as, "Look at the total picture of the nursing home," or "Check out the activity programs," is virtually meaningless. Educated consumers want to know the details: "What should I ask to see?" and "What activities should I be aware of?"

Ideally, you should begin learning about nursing homes before you or a relative needs one. You cannot foresee every emergency admission to or sudden discharge from a hospital, but you can decide that nursing home placement is a topic for research if you are elderly or are responsible for the care of a seventy-five-year-old. By thinking ahead, you can help assure that you will not be forced into a hasty admission to a substandard facility. If you have time to plan ahead, you can discuss nursing homes with friends and neighbors, talk with your primary physician, use this book and other literature, and then consolidate that information so that you can make an intelligent decision when the time comes. If, however, due to illness or emergency, you do not have time for such research, be assured that the information you need is in this book.

The Decision to Look for a Nursing Home

In the beginning of the twentieth century, care of the elderly was provided by family members; a nursing home was sought only when the family found it impossible to care for a relative at home. Since family structures have changed over the years and extended-family living is not as common as in the past, nursing facilities have become a necessary part of the community.

The population aged eighty-five and older is increasing at a spectacular rate, and the nursing home population is likely to grow correspondingly. The U.S. Bureau of the Census reports that in the period between 1980 and 1985, the population aged eighty-five and older increased by 21 percent—from 2.24 million to 2.71 million. At that rate of increase, the number will reach 4.9 million by the year 2000 and will soar to 7.1 million by 2020.

The National Center for Health Statistics indicates there were 1.5 million nursing home residents living in the nation's 19,100 nursing homes and related facilities in 1985. According to the center's survey, if the same rates of dependency continue, the number of elderly living in nursing homes will increase to 3.1 million by 2025. In 1989, there were approximately 15,900 nursing homes certified to participate in the Medicare and Medicaid programs, the highest number of which were in California, Texas, and Ohio and the lowest number in Washington, D.C. and Alaska. In 1990, it is estimated that there were over 21,000 nursing homes, including those not participating in the federally funded programs of Medicare and/or Medicaid, and more facilities are being built every day.

The nursing home population at any one time is a very small percentage of the elderly; less than 5 percent according to the National Center for Health Statistics. Of the population aged sixty-five to seventy-four, less than 1.5 percent are in nursing homes at any one time, but over 20 percent of the population aged eighty-five years and older are receiving nursing home care. Researchers have documented that approximately one in every four elderly people will use a nursing home before they die, and if you are living alone and in a cold-weather state you are probably at a greater risk of needing nursing home care than if you live in the South.

The annual-cost history of nursing home care has been $30 billion, including federal, state, and private spending. Medicaid spends more than $14 billion yearly, and Medicare, about $650 million on nursing home care, while private insurance covers only about 1 percent of long-term care costs.

Most nursing home residents are widowed females. Cognitive impairment, such as occurs in Alzheimer's disease and mental illness, is one of the primary reasons for admissions to nursing homes. Other causative diseases include emphysema, heart disease, stroke, Parkinson's disease, cancer, kidney disorders, and AIDS.

It is important to remember that not all people seventy-five or older are candidates for nursing homes. I have a ninety-five-year-old grandmother who is still living at home and taking care of herself with only minimal family help. But what if you suspect that your relative, regardless of age, *does* need nursing home care? How do you begin to talk about this, and what factors are there to consider? Who will pay for care? Can someone be made to go to a nursing home if he refuses? These are just some of the questions families ask.

If you talk to your relative about the subject, he may become very upset. He may tell you that he is perfectly content living where he is, whether this be in his own home or with you. However, there are many factors to consider beside contentment. Is he functioning independently, or does he need constant supervision for safety reasons? Does he sit alone for hours, perhaps in the dark, forgetting to turn on the lights? One friend told me he knew the time had come to look at nursing homes when his mother began refusing meals, saying, "I'm not hungry." She would sit in front of the television for hours and get up only to go to bed. She was becoming increasingly unkempt in her personal appearance, would wander out of doors alone in the middle of the night, and forget to turn off the stove. Here was a formerly active woman who had taken pride in her appearance and loved preparing meals. Now she was losing weight and refusing to have dinner with the family. She would become argumentative and hostile toward family members when they suggested helping with her personal care.

Even if your relative does not want to talk to you about nursing homes, the truth may be that he can no longer function independently, tends to sit alone for hours, and needs twenty-four hour supervision. Perhaps your relative doesn't engage in conversation or participate in activities he previously enjoyed, becomes depressed and despondent, demonstrates a lack of concern for personal hygiene, experiences periods of sleeplessness or loss of appetite and weight, or refuses to see friends, stating that he has nothing in common with them anymore. He may be unable to concentrate on reading a book or newspaper, or he may lose control of his bladder and bowel. These are just a few of the things that you may notice in your relative and they are all very personal.

He may feel that you are invading his privacy even by broaching the issue and may become very upset, attempting to justify and rationalize his actions by saying, "I sleep so much because there's nothing to do here!" In reality, he is probably feeling boxed in, for he cannot meet what he feels are your expectations of him. He may know that his memory is beginning to fail him, but by admitting it to you, he feels defeated. He wants to maintain his independence and feeling of self-worth, but how can he do this and still admit to you that he is misplacing objects, losing his train of thought, and feeling nervous and anxious over every little thing?

If your relative is living with you, it may be that providing ongoing care has become too overwhelming for you emotionally, physically, and economically. The risks of having him continue to live in this way are grave indeed, both to him and to you and your family. Factors such as wandering, incontinence, and unsafe smoking habits may be extremely difficult to control in a family environment. Cases similar to the following one are not uncommon.

S.B. was an unmarried sixty-eight-year-old living with her ninety-two-year-old mother. S.B. was in charge of all household chores and expenses. For two years she had been caring for her mother at home, taking her to and from the doctor. Her mother had become increasingly disoriented and had even wandered out of the house unsupervised. She had left pots unattended on a hot stove and had almost caused a fire by careless smoking. She became very angry when S.B. suggested household help, and she refused to let anyone in to take care of her.

S.B. had recently found out that she herself had lung cancer. She was becoming weaker and required many rest periods during the day. She could neither supervise her mother's activities nor tend to the household chores as carefully as she would have liked. Attempts at home care had been unsuccessful. S.B. and her mother had no one to depend on, so S.B.'s physician suggested a nursing home for her mother.

With the help of her doctor, S.B. was able to place her mother in a nursing facility near their home. She then hired a part-time companion to help her with household work. Since S.B. had no relatives or friends close by, she knew that in the future she, too, would need the care that only a nursing home could give.

Shortly after her mother's admission to the nursing home, S.B. suffered from insomnia, restlessness, and long periods of depression. Her doctor diagnosed her as having a reactive depression brought on by months of stress and fatigue in caring for her elderly mother.

Had S.B. prepared herself by consulting her doctor and/or a geriatric social worker at an earlier date, she might have been saved some of the anxiety and mental suffering that accompanied placing her mother in a nursing home.

Of course, not all elderly people who are confused need nursing home care. Infections, vitamin deficiencies, thyroid disorders, and liver disease can cause confusion and disorientation. A thorough physical examination is always necessary as a preliminary diagnostic tool in determining the necessity of nursing home placement.

Another frequently asked question is the one my neighbor asked me: "Can I admit my father to a nursing home even if he refuses to go? He is very alert but is constantly demanding of my family's and my time. He becomes hostile and fights with us when we try to help him with his bath and his needs. We have never enjoyed a close relationship, and now that he lives with me we are constantly on each other's nerves. He gets very confused at times and no other living arrangement has worked out."

Some families are under the misconception that they can decide when and if it is time to put a relative into a nursing home; however, there is no such thing as an involuntary admission to a nursing home. An individual alone is responsible for his own welfare as long as he is competent. Only if a resident is adjudicated incompetent or unable to communicate with others can someone else act in his best interest. Usually that person is the next of kin or appointed guardian. When mental competence is in question, a physician or a geriatric evaluation team, consisting of physicians, social workers, and nurses, may have to be consulted regarding nursing home admission.

In my neighbor's case, the family doctor determined that her father was competent but was suffering from many stresses. He suggested family counseling and when this failed to alleviate the problems, the doctor suggested a group home for her father. The family was fortunate to find a good home close by, and her father is now content living with others his own age. Group living was the answer for this family but is not always the solution for everyone.

Another friend asked if her aunt, recently diagnosed with a mental illness, could be admitted to a nursing home. In the past, some patients suffering from mental illness were placed in nursing homes—hence the reputation of some nursing homes as "mental institutions." New federal regulations require pre-admission screening of prospective residents who are exhibiting signs and symptoms of mental illness, to ensure that nursing home beds will not be used for those in need of intense psychiatric care.

What about the person of sound mind, living alone with no family to counsel him, who must make a decision about alternate living arrangements? The following story illustrates the dimensions of this situation.

For some time, R.W. had felt his memory failing on topics with which he had always been familiar. Then there was that incident in which he found himself on the floor in the bathroom and could not recall how he had gotten there. He was also feeling a little weaker as he carried out his daily activities and had no one who could help him on a daily basis.

And was it yesterday or last week that someone had offered him a hand at the grocery store because he'd stumbled—over nothing, but nevertheless had lost his footing? Oh, it had seemed like such a struggle to make it home again! He had heard of such things as strokes happening to older people—but not to him! His blood pressure was normal, or so he thought, even though he hadn't seen a doctor in months. When he finally went to the doctor, he found that his blood pressure was alarmingly high, one kidney was failing, and his reflexes were very sluggish. He had fallen several times and could not remember what caused the falls. The doctor was aware that this gentleman was living alone with no family or close friends.

It was the doctor's decision to broach the subject of a nursing home to R.W., hoping that the gentleman would realize that the time for nursing home care was approaching and that if he waited, he could very well find himself prostrate on the street rather than on the bathroom floor. He gently sat R.W. down and talked to him. The man was sad, but knew the doctor was right. An admission to a nursing home was planned.

Using This Book

How to Choose a Nursing Home: A Guide to Quality Caring shows you how to evaluate nursing homes and choose the one that most closely fits your needs. It can help you in your search for long-term care, because I have seen first hand what works. I've also experienced what doesn't work.

When it came time to take my father to a nursing home, I did not know as much as I do today. I was beset with feelings of anxiety, guilt, and inadequacy. I experienced frequent crying spells and insomnia. My father had always been there, taking care and watching over me, and now I was deserting him when he needed me most. After much consulting with our family physician, I decided that a nursing home was the only solution. I mistakenly chose one for the wrong reason—because it was close to our home. It was also very expensive, but my reasoning then was, "You get what you pay for." However, behind all the expensive furniture and fixtures was an uncaring, unprofessional, and overworked staff. After much distress and concern, we decided to transfer him to another nursing home with which we were all pleased. Here the staff treated him with respect and compassion which helped him regain his self-esteem and maintain his dignity.

In this book you will learn about all aspects of nursing homes. The first two chapters will give you basic information about how nursing homes operate. Chapter 3 will show you, step by step, how to find a nursing home that can offer your relative a high quality of care. You'll learn what to look for when you make comparison visits to nursing homes and how to evaluate what you observe. Chapter 4 will explain how to pay for nursing home care and Chapter 5 will tell you about the move to a nursing home: what to bring, what to leave at home, and what to expect. Chapter 6 is based on hundreds of discussions I've had with residents' families about a wide variety of medical, social, and emotional issues. In this question-and-answer chapter, I will tell you about families' most common concerns. In Chapter 7, you will learn how to handle nursing home problems effectively. Chapter 8 fully discusses the difficult subject of dying in a nursing home. Finally, since I believe that citizen activism is a major route to improving the care in nursing homes, I have concluded this book with an afterword on citizen and government involvement. The greatest influence on the quality of life in nursing homes results from the efforts of advocacy groups for the elderly.

I have chosen to simplify the reading and writing of this book by referring to both residents and nursing home employees as "he" in one chapter and "she" in the next, alternating throughout. The exceptions are in Chapter 6, where the questions and answers refer to both sexes, and in the real-life case histories and examples that appear throughout.

The book speaks primarily to family members who are placing an elderly relative in a nursing home. However, all of the information applies as well to readers who are looking for placement for themselves. The term "nursing home," rather than "nursing center" or "rehabilitative center," is used throughout the book because it is more familiar.

The case histories and individual situations have been gathered from my own and my co-workers' experiences. Families and friends offered suggestions, but most importantly, residents themselves contributed through their daily activities and conversations.

I decided not to discuss alternative living situations in detail, since my own experience is chiefly with nursing homes. However, I urge you to explore any alternatives that seem appropriate for your situation: day care and senior citizen centers, family support centers, homemaker services and agencies, sheltered housing, hospice care, homes and apartments for senior citizens, shared or group housing, visiting nurse services, home health aides, companions, and volunteer services. Many services, including legal advice, telephone programs, senior transportation programs, and mental health projects make it easier for the elderly to live full and productive lives in the community, assured of guidance and protection. You can contact your local Office of Consumer Affairs, the National Council on Aging, or a hospital social worker for more information on these. In addition, the local library is an excellent source of publications on alternative living situations for the elderly. The National Institute on Aging publishes a booklet entitled "Self-Care and Self-Help Groups for the Elderly: A Directory" (#84-738, 1984) which they will send to you.

Appendix A of *How to Choose a Nursing Home: A Guide to Quality Caring* contains a nursing home resident's Bill of Rights. This Bill of Rights, which according to federal regulations must be posted in each nursing facility, deals with the safety, well-being, and privacy of each individual in a nursing home. Residents, visitors, and families should continually refer to it when questioning various aspects of an individual's rights. It is probably the single most important document to consider when asking yourself if a nursing home offers a high quality of life.

Appendix B is a directory that lists each state's director on aging. You can contact your state's agency on aging when you have complaints about a specific nursing home.

Appendix C lists, region by region, the directors of the state departments responsible for the licensing and certification of health facilities. You can call on these agencies when you want to register a complaint about a nursing home.

Various resource centers are mentioned throughout this book, and their addresses are listed alphabetically in Appendix D. I urge you to call on these agencies for information or help with problems. Appendix E is a list of the medications most commonly given to geriatric patients. The list includes most of the widely used drugs, but is not complete, since new medications are constantly being introduced.

After the appendices, I have included a glossary of medical terms for quick reference. Nothing is more annoying than to receive a bill written in medical hieroglyphics and have to decipher its meaning. For additional information on terminology, refer to a standard medical reference (such as *Dorland's Illustrated Medical Dictionary* or *Stedman's Medical Dictionary*) at your local library.

This book is intended to be a comprehensive guide to nursing homes. You may already have heard of another consumer guidebook published by the Health Care Financing Administration. It is based upon past survey and inspection reports of nursing homes and gives statistical profiles of residents. However, I caution you to use this government publication very carefully. While it can be helpful as another source of information in your search for a nursing home, the reports in it are already dated, and conditions in nursing homes change over a period of time. My book offers you personal advice and discusses various solutions to problems you may experience. It also tells you about survey reports and how they affect a nursing home's reputation.

As you read this book, keep in mind that each person is an individual; what works in one case may not work in another. I hope that, by sharing my experiences, I can make your search for high quality of care—what it is and what it isn't—simpler and more successful. Modern nursing homes should offer more than medical services; they should be homes where the elderly can continue, as much as possible, to live lives of dignity and meaning—where caregiving is based upon an individual's needs, not on the needs of the facility.

I have many fond memories of residents, but one that is especially dear to me is of a poet-patient, Mr. Robert H. Davidson, who lived his final days at the nursing home to the fullest, sharing his poems and experiences with those around him. From the moment this gentleman entered our building he became an inspiration to everyone. Even now, I can smell the aroma of his pipe smoke as he sat and spoke of his past with us, reciting lines from his poem, "friendship making the world do what he wills." He was the picture of happiness and serenity and conveyed these feelings in his poem written in 1972:

Who said that love is but a fleeting thing
And years together only dullness bring?
How wrong, how wrong, to make so base a claim
For he who makes it has himself to blame.
Thank God for all the love-filled years
So full of joy, with little left for tears.

Not only did he experience the highest quality of life, but he added much to the lives of those around him.

1

How Nursing Homes Are Regulated

To choose a nursing home that is concerned with the quality of its residents' lives, you have to know what you are looking for. The care of the elderly and infirm is complex, and as a layperson, you may not always be aware of what is involved. For instance, common sense may tell you to check the cleanliness of each facility and the pleasantness of the staff, but would you think to ask about the labeling of medications or the prevention and treatment of pressure sores? Would you think to ask if your relative's funds are kept separate from other residents' funds? And if her funds, kept at the nursing home, are available to her at all times?

Fortunately, you do not have to learn about every aspect of care to judge a nursing home adequately. Federal and state inspectors do the groundwork for you, visiting and evaluating nursing homes and publishing reports you can obtain. This chapter will tell you about the kinds of nursing homes that inspectors look at, the minimum standards that nursing homes are expected to meet, why inspection reports are sometimes flawed, where you can find reports on nursing homes, and what "substandard nursing home" means.

How Nursing Homes Are Classified

Although we tend to discuss nursing homes as though they were all alike, there are actually four distinct categories of nursing homes. The distinction between the classifications is made by federal agencies, but the states license the nursing home for various levels of intensity of care such as personal care (domiciliary), intermediate, skilled, or multilevel. Each type, until recently, provided a different level of intensity of care, had different staffing requirements, and was evaluated by state and federal inspectors according to separate standards. According to the Nursing Home Reform Law, as part of the 1987 Omnibus Budget Reconciliation Act (OBRA), the distinction between a skilled and intermediate facility was eliminated and all skilled and intermediate nursing homes, as of October 1990, were classified under one title: "nursing facility."

The new federal and state regulations required many changes in staffing, training of nursing assistants, and development of procedures and plans. These changes were implemented at various approved time intervals, and by October 1990, both skilled and intermediate facilities as "nursing facilities" were required to comply with the same regulations.

A nursing home meeting the federal regulations may receive federal funding for its residents' care. These nursing homes, when approved, are federally "certified" to participate in the Medicare and Medicaid programs. The nursing home must have annual and follow-up inspections to receive its "recertification," which is based upon compliance with federal and state regulations. If you wish, you can obtain a copy of your state's rules and regulations through your state's licensing and certification department (see Appendix C).

Because you will choose a nursing home based primarily on the type of care you or your family member needs, it is important for you to know the differences between the kinds of nursing homes, especially if you have a relative who has been in a nursing home prior to the new October 1990 classification of "nursing facility."

Personal Care Nursing Homes

A personal care (domiciliary or room and board) home provides a limited amount of care and supervision for those who need less care than in a nursing home. These homes are not always staffed with licensed nurses as many of them are actually part of the owner's home. There are no federal regulations for personal care homes but they are usually licensed by the state. They are less expensive than nursing homes since they do not provide medical care.

Intermediate Care Nursing Homes

An intermediate care facility (ICF) is for residents who need more than room and board but do not need specialized or intensive care. Instead, they need health-related services. Some of the services provided at an ICF are the administration of medications, special diets, and assistance in the activities of daily living as directed by a physician's plan of care.

There is another type of intermediate facility known as ICF-MR for those who are classified as needing intermediate care but whose diagnosis is mental retardation.

Skilled Care Nursing Homes

Another type of nursing home, a skilled nursing facility (SNF), also follows a physician-directed written plan of care for each individual resident. However, an SNF offers a more intensive level of care than an ICF and is equipped and staffed to provide treatments such as sophisticated drugs, inhalation and intravenous therapy, and tube feedings. Residents in an SNF may be in need of a registered physical, occupational, or speech therapist to restore lost function and provide rehabilitation. Some residents may be receiving intensive treatment for skin disorders, such as skin ulcers, and others may be victims of AIDS or require constant supervision because of dementia-related behavior.

Multilevel Nursing Homes

Multilevel nursing homes have both intermediate and skilled beds available, either on the same unit or on separate floors or "wings."

By late 1990, OBRA legislation required that all "nursing facilities" be staffed with licensed nurses twenty-four hours a day and use a registered, professional nurse on the day tour of duty seven days a week.

Chronic Care Facilities

There is another type of facility in some states called a chronic disease facility (hospital). The chronic disease facility provides care for the most seriously ill—typically people who have suffered a massive stroke, are in the last stages of a terminal disease, or have had serious injuries due to accidents. A much wider range of services and a higher ratio of nurses to patients is available in a chronic facility than in the other two types of nursing homes.

A chronic care facility is equipped to handle the care of a resident in need of rehabilitation from conditions such as neurologic disease, strokes, or multiple fractures. In addition, patients with chronic diseases such as multiple sclerosis may benefit from the services available at a chronic care facility. The goal of a chronic care facility is to meet the needs of residents who require more complex care with special equipment and provide services not usually available in a nursing home, in the hopes that a resident can someday be moved to another, less intensive-care living arrangement. When this is not possible (as may happen in the case of a patient with terminal cancer), the goal becomes the provision of needed care. Some states do not have chronic care facilities, so services that would normally be offered at a chronic care facility are rendered at a hospital.

When you are checking regulations on licensing of nursing homes, you will find that licensing criteria differs from state to state, as well as the number of skilled, intermediate, and/or chronic facilities. And since cost is always an important consideration when looking at nursing homes, you should know that an ICF is generally the least expensive type of nursing home and a chronic care facility is usually the most expensive. However, the extra services and treatments required by a resident are the major determinants of the total cost of care.

As you look at the various types of nursing homes, you may hear two descriptive terms: proprietary and nonproprietary. These words do not refer to levels of care in nursing homes but rather to ownership. Proprietary nursing homes are operated for profit. Nonproprietary nursing homes are usually affiliated with religious, governmental, or fraternal organizations and are not for profit.

A final word on classifications as you begin to look at nursing homes. Some homes accept private pay patients only and are not certified to receive federal or state funding. There could be several reasons for this. Some owners claim they accept only private paying residents and thereby eliminate all the paperwork and "red tape" required by the government. Others say that federal funds are not enough to provide care to the residents. Be particularly cautious when looking at facilities not certified to receive federal and state funds. The reason some of these homes are not licensed and certified is because of the poor quality of care they provide! If in doubt, check with the various resource centers listed in Appendix D.

What Inspectors Look For

According to state and federal regulations, nursing homes are subject to unannounced annual and follow-up inspections. At the time of the surveys, government inspectors (also called surveyors or auditors) come with questions and forms, and spend several days checking on all aspects of patient care and quality of life components. They review the residents' records and compare their observations and interviews against the documentation. If you have a basic understanding of what inspectors look for, you will gain some insight into the working of a nursing home and be better able to interpret the published inspection reports about the nursing homes you are considering.

Nursing home inspectors are concerned with both the physical and emotional care of residents. As they enter a room they may observe a bed-confined resident who is not in a comfortable position. She may be lying in a bed with the side rails down (a safety hazard) or she may be crying out to use a bedpan. The inspectors may even hear a radio blaring loud music of the staff's choice, or detect strong, unpleasant smells in the resident's room.

They may find a resident who has a bedsore that developed in the nursing home. They will check the resident's records to determine what methods and treatments were used by the staff to try to prevent the bedsore. A friend told me the following story about a survey held while she was visiting her mother.

The surveyors walked in and found food plates uncovered and the food served at unsafe and unpalatable temperatures. When they walked into Mother's room, they found she was not prepared for her meal. Mother was not sitting up, didn't have her dentures, and her clothing was not protected against food spills and stains. They checked the dishes and flatware and found them chipped and stained.

The surveyors will also check diet cards on the residents' trays and compare their diet to the doctor's orders. They may find that a facility provides excellent care in all other aspects but must improve in carrying out the doctor's dietary orders.

They review medical records to ensure family members have been called when a resident's health status has changed.

The timeliness of administration of medications is reviewed during the inspection process and the nurse is carefully watched as she prepares the medicines.

During the inspection process, surveyors routinely interview from 10 to 20 percent of the residents, depending on the size of the nursing home. Each resident is asked questions concerning her care and needs and whether they are met agreeably. For instance, if a surveyor finds a plate of food left uncovered for a long time and sees that the resident is not eating, she may ask the resident if the food is tasty and why she is not eating.

Complaint logs are reviewed, and since resident councils are active in the presentation of residents' grievances, surveyors talk with council representatives to ensure that the residents' individual grievances are addressed without recrimination. They then determine if the staff has provided timely follow-ups and corrections to identified problems or grievances.

One resident told a surveyor that bedspreads in the nursing home were old and needed replacing. She had asked the laundry department about new ones and nothing was ever done. "I brought up the subject at a resident meeting and the council followed through to make sure we got new spreads."

In an interview with a resident, a surveyor may notice that she appears depressed. The surveyor checks the resident's record to see if depression was a problem before admission, when it was first noted, and the treatment, if any, that the resident has been receiving for her depression. She determines if the problem has been adequately assessed and documented, with measurable goals and outcomes on the resident's plan of care. Other problems that are checked in this way are infections, insomnia, inappropriate behavior, and loss of weight.

During their inspection, surveyors will talk to the nursing assistants and will ask them questions about the residents. They may ask the diagnosis, the therapies a resident is attending, and the foods the patient likes and dislikes. They observe the assistant while she provides daily care to the resident. They watch as the resident is moved from her bed to a chair and note whether safety devices are being used when necessary.

Surveyors are also concerned with the environmental condition of the nursing home and the efficiency of its operations.

Since OBRA provides for posting of survey results in nursing homes as of October 1990, the surveyors check to see that the results of the most recent survey are accessible to both residents and families.

EXAMPLES OF QUESTIONS INSPECTORS ASK

- Are residents free from mental/physical abuse?
- Are restraints used only on doctors' orders?
- Are residents informed of their rights?
- Are physicians notified promptly of test results?
- Are families notified promptly of a resident's injury?
- Are residents treated with dignity?
- Do residents participate in the planning of their care?
- Do residents have choices in schedules and activities?
- Do residents have a homelike environment?
- Are residents notified before a room change is made?
- Is the number and address of the state survey office and ombudsman's office posted for the residents?
- Are the residents' needs being met with the provided staff?

Surveyors ask at least one nurse, or assistant, the procedures to follow in case of fire or other emergency and ask the locations of fire extinguishers.

Infection control is extremely important to the health of the residents. Surveyors will observe staff performance in carrying out infection control measures during the survey.

When you consider that these are just a few items inspectors must check, you can see how complex nursing home care and its evaluation can be. If you examine some of the surveyors' concerns in detail, you will understand why these issues are important to residents and their families.

First, consider the question of a resident's right to participate in her care and to refuse treatment if she desires. A surveyor will check to see that a patient's wishes are not ignored.

I can remember one resident's objections to taking her medication and the reasons she gave.

Mrs. S., an eighty-nine-year-old resident, decided that as long as she was lucid and alert, she would make up her own mind regarding her care. She was told by her physician that her nausea and dizziness were caused by an inner ear disease, for which the doctor prescribed medicine.

After taking this medicine for several days, Mrs. S. complained of severe dryness in her mouth and periods of forgetfulness and listlessness. She stopped taking the medicine, saying, "I would rather have the nausea and dizziness than the side effects of the medicine."

In Mrs. S.'s case another drug was provided that did not cause these side effects. However, the choice to take or not to take the medicine was hers. Nurses may not always agree with the resident's choices, but ultimately, it is the resident's right to refuse treatment.

In another case, a resident quietly insisted she would not be a burden to her family any longer and turned down further treatment.

Ninety-year-old Mrs. K. was transferred to a nearby hospital in acute pain. Upon hearing that she needed emergency surgery, she refused all further treatment. Her question, "Whose life is this anyway?" was a valid one and did not require an answer from the medical staff. The physician agreed that it was indeed her right to refuse surgery and discharged her back to the nursing home. She quietly passed away in her sleep with her family in attendance. We all felt we had let her down by not persuading her to have the necessary surgery, but later we agreed that the decision was hers and no one could make it for her.

Surveyors investigate another area that may surprise you—residents' privacy. Too often, nurses and assistants walk into a room without knocking and otherwise deprive residents of their privacy. The issue of sexuality is also involved here. Mrs. B.'s case was a good example of both privacy and sexuality issues.

> *Every morning, Mrs. B. could be found snuggled up in bed with her husband in his room across the hall. Mr. B.'s condition required that he have a private room or the provision for a double room for the couple would have been made. Mrs. B. would awaken before him, climb out of his bed, cover him with his blanket, and tiptoe out of his room, quietly closing the door behind her. She would cross the hall to her own room and proceed to wash and dress herself for breakfast. For the forty-six years of their marriage Mrs. B. had slept by her husband's side, and she was not about to change her habits just because she was in a nursing home.*

As aging occurs, the sense of touch becomes even more important and special to an individual, conveying feelings of compassion and love. In Mrs. B.'s case, her contact with her husband (physical as well as emotional) kept her from feeling isolated and lonely. She was allowed to exercise her right to privacy and maintain her close relationship with her spouse.

In addition to looking at residents' rights to privacy and participation in their own care, surveyors will check that residents are not transferred or discharged without prior consent of the resident and/or the family or legal guardian.

Another area surveyors check is a nursing home's employment practices, since adequate staffing is essential if residents are to receive quality care. As the investigators talk with employees, they check name tags against the daily attendance record to ensure that the names on the daily work schedule are the names of the employees who are on duty. In years past, to suggest that staffing needs had been met, some nursing homes claimed that certain employees were on the staff when they were not. Individual states vary in their nursing home staffing requirements. Federal regulations require that the nursing home provide nursing services which are sufficient to meet nursing needs of all the residents all hours of each day.

The surveyors check on the availability of social workers, dietitians, physical, occupational, and speech therapists as well as the supplemental services of a dentist and podiatrist. With OBRA's regulations requiring a quality assurance program to be in effect in all nursing homes, the program, if operating effectively, will identify problem areas before they become a major concern. Each nursing home will have a team consisting of various members of the nursing home staff. They will check on each other's departments, responsibilities, and functioning. Forms and reports will be used and problem areas recorded, in much the same way that the surveyors work when they come to the nursing homes. The functioning of the quality assurance team will be checked closely by the surveyors during their inspections.

Another important element of a resident's rights is the one that clarifies a nursing home's requirement to manage a resident's personal funds if and when a resident requests. Management of a resident's funds used to be up to the discretion of the nursing home's administrator until new regulations made it mandatory to help the resident with personal fund management. Surveyors will check to see that the service is provided and that proper records are maintained when assistance is needed.

EXAMPLES OF WHAT INSPECTORS CHECK

- Cleanliness and safety of the building
- Food storage, preparation, and service
- Emergency power supplies
- Proper functioning of call lights
- Accuracy of medication recording
- Room and water temperatures
- Excessive use of tranquilizers
- Fingernails, toenails, hair, teeth, and the personal grooming of the residents
- Provision of rehabilitation services
- Activity programs
- Observation of residents' rights
- Availability of fire extinguishers
- Adequacy of lighting
- Medical records
- Physicians' orders and nurses' documentation

Surveys of a nursing home are complex processes and may leave some of your questions unanswered. Official inspection reports for Medicare and Medicaid certification provide specific information regarding deficiencies found during the survey. However, conditions can improve or deteriorate rapidly when changes take place with key staff

personnel or when a nursing home has financial management difficulties. Nursing homes may seem to comply with
all the written regulations and yet not offer an acceptable
standard of living for you or your relative. You shouldn't
substitute state or federal inspection reports for your own
first-hand look at a nursing home. Rather, you should use
these reports as a starting point for your own investigations.

Public Reports and How to Get Them

When an inspection is over, a surveyor documents,
records, and makes public any problems she has seen. The
Freedom of Information Act ensures public access to these
inspection reports. You can check the results of surveys at
your district Social Security office or by contacting the local
ombudsman's office to receive information on the location
of public disclosures. Several states provide the survey
disclosures in local libraries. Recent Medicare and Medicaid
certification survey reports are to be posted, in an easily
accessible spot, in all nursing homes as of October 1990.
Check these survey reports for any nursing home you are
considering. Keep in mind that even the best nursing homes
may have to correct essential areas of concern when
surveyed. A plan of correction is then submitted by the
facility.

There is another report that might interest you. In 1986,
the Special Committee on Aging, chaired by Senator John
Heinz (R-Pa.), completed a two-year study on intermediate
and skilled nursing homes in the United States. The study
was based on interviews with residents of nursing homes,
personnel in the homes, and inspection reports.

The committee's investigation confirmed that stricter
inspections and enforcement of quality-care laws were
needed to ensure the well-being of our elderly in nursing
homes. The Special Committee reported that the Department of Health and Human Services (DHHS) had failed to
ensure that nursing homes receiving federal funds were
providing the highest quality of care possible. In response to
the report, DHHS drafted a revised—and more stringent—set
of procedures to be used in conducting nursing home
surveys. The implementation of the federal procedures by
the Health Care and Financing Administration (HCFA) began
in July 1986 and is known as the "Long-Term Care Survey
Process" (LTCSP).

The LTCSP guidelines place more emphasis on quality of care and patient outcomes. As a result of these guidelines, surveyors are required to observe the actual daily care, as well as the special treatments and medications, given to individual residents. Although this is a step in the right direction—toward the assessment of the components that add to the quality of life in nursing homes—the HCFA continues to revise survey guidelines to eliminate recurrent evaluation problems.

Substandard Nursing Homes

An example of what a surveyor might observe in a substandard nursing home follows:

It is 7:30 p.m. and Mrs. A. is sitting in the television room, food on the floor in front of her and her supper tray on a nearby table. The furniture is in poor repair, the lighting is dim, and the room is in need of fresh paint. Another resident is sitting nearby, smoking a cigarette, and there is no ventilation. There is a strong unpleasant smell in the room. Two nursing assistants are in the room, talking loudly to each other about their difficult assignments and whose job it is to put Mrs. A. to bed. When Mrs. A. cries out loudly for help, they respond to her in an undignified manner.

This is a scene we hope never to see, yet the Special Committee on Aging reported that some homes are known to be substandard in the care they provide to their residents. Some facilities have the reputation of treating their residents with little dignity and underpaying their staff.

The Special Committee disclosed that, in 1984, one-third of the 8,852 certified skilled nursing facilities failed to meet at least one federal requirement and 11 percent (1,000) failed to meet three or more such requirements. In four recent nationwide on-site inspections, 6.6 percent of skilled facilities were reported to be chronically deficient in the care they provided to residents.

You may wonder if the problems are serious and life-threatening and what causes a nursing home to be chronically deficient. Some of the reported violations involved the following: failure to adequately provide training of nursing home staff; no licenses available for several nurses and/or physical therapists; unacceptable nursing care; and drug carts left unlocked and unprotected.

According to the February 1986 Ombudsman's Summary, the categories of complaints in nursing homes include resident care, food and nutrition, residents' rights, medications, and physician's services.

A typical scene in a chronically deficient nursing home is a resident's room at mealtime.

> *Mrs. W. is lying in bed, unkempt. A lunch tray rests on the bedside stand, no call light is available for her, and soiled dressings lie on her overbed table. A nursing assistant walks in and tells the resident that the nursing home is always short of help and she doesn't have time to help her. As the assistant walks out of the room— without telling the resident whether she'll return—it is obvious that she is lacking in compassion and concern for the well-being of the elderly.*

Another example of chronically substandard conditions is a nursing home whose kitchen equipment is stained and soiled with old food spills, where the serving utensils are unsanitary, and the menus are not served as ordered (such as serving meal trays with sugar on them to diabetic residents). In the same nursing home can be found residents' dentures left on food trays; soiled floors throughout the facility; damaged cabinets, drawers, and closet doors; leaking faucets and unsafe water temperatures. Wheelchairs, geriatric chairs, and other medical equipment in this facility is left unclean, and an inadequate supply of bed linens is evident.

The Special Committee on Aging found conditions like these in substandard nursing homes. The amendments to federal regulations and guidelines brought about by OBRA will help to ensure that such offenses will not be tolerated in nursing homes.

A nursing home is expected to correct all noncompliances. A follow-up survey is conducted to ensure that action has been taken and that the facility conforms to state and federal regulations. However, under federal regulations, a nursing home may continue to receive Medicare and Medicaid funding for a predetermined period of time only if an acceptable plan of correction is provided. A certification agreement is issued, with an automatic cancellation clause to take effect within an agreed-upon time frame, if the outstanding deficiencies are not corrected.

Why should a nursing home be allowed to continue providing care to residents if it has been found noncompliant in some areas? Decertification is the only federal penalty that can be imposed on facilities that do not comply with health standards. Decertification usually results in closing the facility because it cannot continue to function without federal funding. When there is an immediate or serious threat to the health or safety of the residents in a nursing home, the residents must be transferred to other facilities.

Proposed enforcement of OBRA regulations now being finalized by the Health Care Financing Administration will provide stimuli to ensure that nursing homes not only achieve compliance but maintain it as well. Some of the remedies include temporary management, a ban on admissions of residents within certain diagnostic categories, and a ban on payment for new admissions. Additionally, OBRA calls for a directed plan of correction and monitoring by the state. The use of civil money penalties will also be available, but will come under the jurisdiction of the office of the Inspector General. Remedies can delay the termination of the nursing home's participation for no more than six months, during which time payment can continue to the facility despite noncompliances.

This procedure is used for facilities that are substandard but are judged not to be so poor as to require decertification. A nursing home that fails to comply within the required time frame will be terminated from the federally funded programs. When the deficiencies have been corrected, the nursing home can be reinstated into the programs after a required length of time has passed.

If there is an immediate and serious threat to the health or safety of the residents, the Health Care Financing Administration can either terminate the nursing home's participation in the federally funded program or immediately appoint a temporary manager to remove the threat. Other remedies may be imposed, as necessary, to bring the nursing home into full compliance of federal regulations.

Because of the potential problems resulting from changes of key personnel, financial management difficulties, official evaluations, and substandard nursing homes, it is necessary for you to take an active part in judging and choosing a nursing home. One of the most important things to consider is the quality of the staff in a nursing home. The next chapter will tell you what employees should be doing and how to evaluate what you see.

2

How Nursing Homes Operate

Anursing home is as good as the people who work in it. When nursing home staff members come together as a team, doing their jobs in a compassionate and conscientious way, there is a high quality of life for the residents. But if staff members are poorly trained and unmotivated, the quality of life for residents will be poor, even if the nursing home has a modern facility and fine-sounding programs. Because staff members are so important, you need to understand how a nursing home's team *should* function and what each employee *should* be doing. Once you know this, you can visit a nursing home and judge how well the staff performs.

The day-to-day operations of a nursing home are run by three people: the administrator, the medical director, and the director of nurses—all responsible to a policy-making board. These are the people who supervise and set the tone for the nursing home. Under them are all the departments and all the other employees, including the staff members who provide most of the actual care of residents: nursing assistants and orderlies.

WHO IS IN CHARGE?

The Administrator Supervises all staff members and oversees all nursing home operations.

The Medical Director Directs medical care for residents, either personally or through residents' own physicians.

The Director of Nurses Oversees all nursing care and supervises nurses, assistants, and orderlies.

Employees of the different nursing home departments— nursing, dietary, activities, therapies, and social work—hold multidisciplinary meetings to plan the care of each resident. These meetings and the actions that follow them are the keys to quality in a nursing home. When all the staff members do their jobs well, a resident ends up with an individualized plan of care that meets his needs and greatly contributes to the quality of his life.

This chapter will first describe the responsibilities of the people who run a nursing home and then tell you about the rest of the nursing home staff. After that, the chapter will describe how interdisciplinary meetings and plans should work.

Administrator

An effective administrator has to be flexible, intelligent, and caring to deal with his multifaceted job. He must run his nursing home according to government standards and directions from the nursing home's governing board, and he must be compassionate in meeting both residents' and employees' needs.

One of the administrators I admire most is Mr. P. He makes daily visits to the nursing units and speaks with each resident and employee by name. He is aware of and responds to the preferences of all those under his care. Mr. P. also is involved in the planning of social activities and outings for his residents. For example, he held an open art show at the nursing home, invited local artists, and arranged for one of them to give art lessons to the residents. During the annual staff/resident picnic, Mr. P. could be found cooking hotdogs and playing horseshoes with the residents. He is continually finding new ways to humanize the facility by providing more personal and meaningful activities. Once he helped his daughter, a cosmetician, put on a "spa day" at the home. She provided make-up lessons for the women and grooming tips for the men, and everyone had a wonderful day at the spa.

In a smaller facility (fewer than 100 beds), the residents can go directly to the administrator or his representatives for improvements in their living arrangements and conditions. In a larger nursing home (more than 150 beds), the residents may have to go through several people before having a request met by the administrator. I have found most administrators very cooperative about reasonable changes.

Mrs. S. liked wine before her evening meal and wanted to continue this custom in the nursing home. "I'm not ready to give up my social contacts and my cocktail hour just because I'm in here," she said adamantly to Mr. B., the nursing home administrator. Mr. B. set aside a part of the dining area for one hour preceding the evening meal on weekends. Then the nurses obtained a doctor's order for a cocktail for those residents who wanted to participate in this "happy hour."

Administrators are licensed through a state's regulatory agency. In years past it was not uncommon to find administrators who had not received formal training in long-term care, and occasionally one could be found who was not even licensed as an administrator. As the state agencies and the National Association of Boards of Nursing Home Examiners grew more involved, it became evident that there was a need for more qualified administrators. Now, licensed administrators are required to pass examinations.

The high quality of life in a nursing home is often a reflection of the relationship between the administrator and the nursing home staff. It is to him, for instance, that the

---

EXAMPLES OF AN
ADMINISTRATOR'S RESPONSIBILITIES

- Ensures that the physical and mental needs of residents are met
- Ensures the safety and upkeep of the nursing home
- Supervises the staff
- Communicates with residents' families
- Conducts a daily "walk through" inspection
- Oversees the finances of the nursing home
- Maintains a liaison between the governing body and the medical and nursing staff
- Creates an atmosphere of warmth, congeniality, and positive emphasis in the facility
- Meets with the department supervisors on a regular basis to eliminate and correct problems
- Manages the residents' funds

director of nursing turns when he needs support to solve a problem. The loyalty and respect that should define the relationship between the administrator and the nursing department permeate all aspects of nursing home life. You can find out if there is good rapport by asking questions. Have meetings with the administrator and director of nurses together. Ask the nursing staff and the director of nurses if they get administrative support. You'd be surprised how much you'll learn this way, for nursing home staff usually tell about the good as well as the bad.

Medical Director

A licensed nursing home is required to work with a principal physician, called a medical director. He plays an active part in developing the policies of the nursing home and is ultimately responsible for the care given to residents with private physicians. To do his job well, the medical director must be attuned to the older generation, recognizing their needs and possessing a strong desire to treat them as individuals with individual problems.

The medical director should oversee the care all residents receive, even though most residents have their own private physicians. If, as in the following case, a private physician does not deliver adequate care, the medical director must intervene.

Mr. K. was a disoriented resident whose family lived out of town and visited him infrequently. His physician was not attentive to his usually incoherent conversations and never took the time to find out how he was feeling or if he needed anything. After much frustration on the staff's part, the nurses consulted the medical director. He talked with the attending physician, who was surprised to hear that the gentleman could indeed express some coherent thoughts if time and patience were given him.

In another situation, the medical director stepped in after observing an unsatisfactory visit by a private physician.

When the physician came to give his nursing home patient a routine examination, he was unaffected by her complaint of a painful right knee, and reminded her of her age and arthritis. Having told her that, the doctor was out the door in a huff. The medical director overheard the conversation, went into the room, and sat down to listen to the resident's complaints. He found out that earlier in the morning she had fallen, but had not thought her swollen knee was related to the fall. The medical director talked to the attending physician, who ordered X-rays. Much to the physician's surprise, the X-rays confirmed the knee was not only arthritically deformed but also broken!

Another responsibility of the medical director is his correspondence with private physicians who are out of compliance with the nursing home's policies and/or federal regulations. For example, according to federal regulations a resident must be examined by a physician within forty-eight hours of admission unless the examination was done within the previous five days. The medical director might write a letter to a private physician who is out of compliance with regulations in the timeliness of his visit to a resident. The medical director also helps decide whether a particular patient should be seen by his private physician every thirty days or less frequently.

Since the medical director oversees the care in a nursing home, he helps set the tone for the residents' quality of life. An effective director is familiar with nursing policies and is available for emergencies twenty-four hours a day. Beyond that, he knows the nursing staff by name, especially the director of nurses and charge nurses on each unit. When you visit a nursing home, ask the nurses if their medical director knows them, and if he knows who runs each unit. Is he familiar with the daily routines on the units? Does he stop to ask the nurses of any concerns they might have? You will quickly find out whether the director takes his responsibility seriously or performs his job in name only.

Director of Nurses

The director of nurses is a registered nurse who is licensed by the state and may have a bachelor's or master's degree in nursing. He is hired by the administrator and is employed full-time. The entire service department is under his direction.

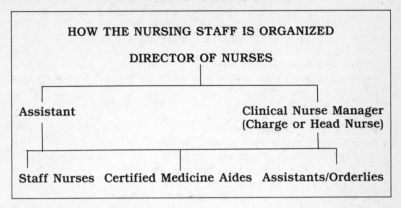

HOW THE NURSING STAFF IS ORGANIZED

DIRECTOR OF NURSES

Assistant

**Clinical Nurse Manager
(Charge or Head Nurse)**

Staff Nurses   Certified Medicine Aides   Assistants/Orderlies

To be effective, the director of nurses must be assertive yet diplomatic, since his duties include supervising staff and communicating with doctors, families, and residents. He should possess good leadership qualities and be able to make requests through the administrator that will benefit the nursing home and improve the residents' quality of life.

One head nurse I knew, Mrs. S., was able to gain the administrator's cooperation in bringing community groups to provide companionship for the residents. High school students, scout troops, and neighborhood children were called by Mrs. S. to help in the nursing home.

She arranged for the activities director to provide cookies and milk and little incentives for those who came to read to the residents. Some of the children she recruited would write letters; others would water the residents' flowers or help with fresh ice and water. Others just sat quietly and provided companionship to those who had no family.

One of the most important responsibilities of the director of nurses is to interpret and clarify doctors' orders when needed. For instance, the director will notify a doctor about a resident's needs or help a charge nurse understand an order that may be confusing.

The director of nurses usually has an assistant, but this is not always the case. The need for an assistant is directly related to the number of residents in the facility and the levels of care that are provided. Sometimes an assistant director may also do in-service training of nursing assistants.

EXAMPLES OF THE
DIRECTOR OF NURSES' RESPONSIBILITIES

- Makes daily rounds to all units
- Supervises, schedules, and evaluates all nurses and assistants
- Reviews the residents' care
- Confers with private doctors and the medical director
- Handles complaints and problems
- Ensures adequate staffing
- Directs and supervises in-service programs
- May help in developing a written plan of care for each resident
- Develops and implements the nursing policies
- Ensures the residents' rights to fair treatment
- Maintains the privacy of each individual resident

Clinical Nurse Manager
(Charge or Head Nurse)

A clinical nurse manager, called a charge or head nurse in some nursing homes, runs one unit or section of the nursing home. The nurse may be a registered nurse (RN) or, in some smaller nursing homes, a licensed practical nurse (LPN). Since continuity and high-quality nursing care are priorities, the charge nurse should be working full-time and be on the staff of the home rather than a temporary agency nurse who is working part-time. While there are many dedicated temporary nurses, an agency nurse cannot offer the continuity of care that elderly residents need. Imagine how confusing it would be to an elderly person to have a different nurse on each shift every day. The inconsistencies of temporary nurses can increase a resident's confusion and leave him feeling insecure. He may ask himself, "Who will be my nurse tonight and tomorrow?" "Will this nurse care about me or will I be just a number in room 3B?"

It takes a nurse with special interest in the problems of the elderly to work as a charge nurse. He deals with the same residents daily, sometimes for months or years, and may see little change in their daily routines. This is not to say that some hospital nurses cannot care for the elderly in the same way a geriatric nurse does. However, the type of patient, the medications, and the routines involved make it necessary for a charge nurse to be familiar with the elderly and their needs.

A conscientious geriatric nurse continually reviews and revises the activity levels of his residents. For example, if you observe a nursing home on a warm and pleasant day, you may find a conscientious charge nurse gathering the residents to go outside for an iced-tea social or an outing in the sun. You may find him participating in the activities program to help stimulate the interest of a group. Such activities require an interested, motivated person, one who is concerned with the quality of the elderly residents' lives.

EXAMPLES OF THE
CLINICAL NURSE MANAGER'S RESPONSIBILITIES

- Directs the unit's nursing services
- Makes rounds of the residents on the unit
- Monitors the residents' medication, diet, and treatment
- Notifies doctors and families as needed
- Ensures cleanliness and infection control on the unit
- Develops a written plan of care for each resident according to the physician's plan of care
- Ensures twenty-four hour nursing services
- Provides ongoing training of nursing assistants
- Maintains a liaison between the family, staff, and residents
- Maintains the privacy of each individual resident

Certified Medicine Aide

In years past it was not unusual to find the charge nurse not only directing the management of the nursing unit but also giving medications and doing the treatments of the residents as required. An exemplary nursing home will hire a specially trained person, or a professional nurse, to give medications. The certified medicine aide (CMA) need not be a licensed nurse but he must complete a special training course on medications and their effects on the elderly. The CMA is certified to give oral medications but a licensed nurse is responsible for any injectable medicines or narcotics.

EXAMPLES OF THE
CMA'S RESPONSIBILITIES

- Prepares and administers medications as ordered by the physician
- Records the residents' blood pressure, temperature, pulse, and respirations when necessary (some medications are not given if the blood pressure and/or pulse are not within normal limits)
- Assists in the residents' nursing care
- Maintains the stock supply of medications
- Checks labels of medications for expiration dates
- Ensures the safe storage of medications
- Maintains the privacy of each individual resident

Geriatric Nursing Assistant

An essential member of the nursing home team is the geriatric nursing assistant (or orderly). Most of the hands-on nursing care is provided by nursing assistants, and until the nursing home reform act the training program for an assistant was not extensive. No regulations ensured that a nursing assistant would be adequately trained prior to actual patient care. Until now, the nursing assistant may have been previously trained or he may have come to the nursing home as an unskilled worker. If an untrained assistant was hired, a course was given by the nursing home, and on-the-job teaching was provided as an ongoing experience by the in-service director and charge nurse.

Legislation has been passed in response to the Institute of Medicine's suggestion that more extensive training of nursing assistants be given. As of October 1, 1990 it became mandatory that nursing assistants be specifically trained and take a state-approved course. Nursing assistants employed in nursing homes before that date will also be evaluated and assessed. This program is another step toward ensuring that a nursing home provide quality care.

It is impossible to list the many and important duties of a nursing assistant, for he is the person who provides most of the hands-on care of the residents. Some of the major responsibilities follow.

EXAMPLES OF THE NURSING ASSISTANT'S RESPONSIBILITIES

- Assists residents with all aspects of daily life
- Provides special services, such as blood pressure reading, enemas, and bladder training programs
- Supervises dining area and mealtime
- Transfers residents for activities, rehabilitation, tests, and hospital stays
- Monitors the residents' health and reports problems to nurses
- Helps the residents to choose activities
- Provides ice water and nourishments to residents
- Makes frequent rounds of the unit to ensure the residents' safety
- Makes rounds with the oncoming shift
- Helps to improve or maintain the residents' physical functioning
- Provides emotional and psychological support
- Maintains the privacy of each individual resident

When a resident has been ordered to remain in bed, it is the nursing assistant who provides his care and meets his nursing needs. He bathes, dresses, and feeds the resident as necessary. He provides extra fluids, monitors his vital signs, maintains a toileting schedule, and generally oversees his total care. He assists the nurse in turning and positioning the resident to maintain good body alignment, supports the resident when he is anxious and allays his fears during uncomfortable treatments, reads to him, makes phone calls for him, and holds his hand when he is in pain and feels alone. He informs the charge nurse of any unusual signs or symptoms and maintains the resident's confidentiality at all times.

Because of the close relationship that develops between the assistant and the resident, the assistant is vulnerable to the resident's quickly changing moods. If he is known to be an excellent care-giver, he will remain calm and emotionally in control as well as amenable to the resident's requests. Daily the nursing assistant faces sickness and death but is expected to do so with a smile on his face, uncomplaining and eager to please.

A nursing assistant is generally considered to be grossly underpaid. The salary of nursing assistants and orderlies is not commensurate with the responsibility of dealing with the everyday issues of life. As one nursing assistant so aptly said, "It never ceases to amaze me that undertakers and morticians receive higher salaries for taking care of the dead than I do for taking care of the living!" Because of the poor compensation and the tiring working conditions, the turnover rate and absenteeism of nursing assistants is high.

Social Worker

The social service director is responsible for the emotional and social needs of individual residents and acts as a liaison between the staff, family, and community services. Under the regulations of OBRA, a nursing home with more than 120 beds will have at least one full-time social worker on staff. He should provide support and help to residents who have any emotional problems or special difficulties, such as financial crises or acute illness.

For example, a social worker discusses with residents and their families the difficult decisions a resident must make, such as the use of life-support systems, if and when these become necessary. If a resident is competent and alert, he will make the decision for himself. However, if he is incompetent or determined by his physician to be incapable of understanding his rights and responsibilities, the social worker will discuss the subject with the resident's next of kin or the resident's representative.

**EXAMPLES OF THE
SOCIAL WORKER'S RESPONSIBILITIES**

- Meets with prospective residents and their families
- Takes families on tours of the nursing home
- Suggests rooms and roommates for prospective residents
- Assesses the physical, emotional, and spiritual needs of the residents
- Encourages family involvement and participation in residents' lives after admission
- Leads small discussion groups with families, residents, and staff
- Plans discharges and suggests community agencies for continuing home care
- Maintains the privacy of each individual resident

The social worker must be extremely tactful and empathetic. He should be soft-spoken and have a calming effect on those around him. His skills as a communicator are very important and he should possess the ability to reduce greatly the stress levels that are present in nursing homes.

In the nursing home where I worked, the social worker spent an entire day sitting with a sick patient, refusing to leave him alone because his family was out of town and not available. This social worker seemed to know intuitively how to allay fear and anxiety. He was the hope of those who felt beyond all hope. When shifts in environment occurred, it was the social worker who came running to the rescue.

Activities Director

It takes an understanding, trained person to create and direct an effective activities program. The director has to set goals, structure a program to meet the needs of a broad range of residents, and run the program efficiently and calmly. He is further challenged because in a nursing home, not only oriented and alert residents take part in activity groups, but also those residents who are less oriented and competent.

There are also those who, due to their medical condition, have given up hope of ever doing anything constructive again. That was true of K.B., before Bob, a young, energetic, and compassionate activities director came to talk to her about her previous interest in sewing.

K.B. was a sixty-year-old woman terminally ill with cancer. The cancerous growth had invaded her cheekbone and her face had become disfigured by numerous treatments. It was becoming very difficult to interest her in any activities, even bathing and dressing. She was very talented at sewing and she had once made all her own clothes. She would smile as she recalled how proud she had been to display her own creations to her friends. With the activities director's help, K.B.'s interest in sewing was rekindled. What a thrill it was when K.B. asked if we could put on a fashion show in which she and other residents would model clothing. It was a very exciting moment when K.B. walked into the room modeling her originally designed jumpsuit!

All programs are subject to a physician's orders. Usually, activities are grouped according to levels of difficulty and may be referred to as Group I, II, III, and IV, or by various colors, such as Red, Green, Blue, and Yellow Group, etc. The activity director tracks residents' activity levels, identifies problems related to the activity program of an individual resident, and records his observations and recommendations on the resident's chart.

EXAMPLES OF THE
ACTIVITIES DIRECTOR'S RESPONSIBILITIES

- Assesses the residents' physical abilities under the direction of the nurse and plans activities accordingly
- Plans social outings, parties, and games
- Takes part in organizing volunteer groups
- Helps to enhance the residents' sense of self-esteem by encouraging participation in group activities
- Maintains a safe and productive activity room
- Visits with residents on a one-to-one basis when they are not able to attend activities
- Respects the residents' wishes and maintains their privacy

Therapists

Nursing homes generally have three kinds of therapists: occupational therapists, physical therapists, and speech therapists. These three kinds of therapists provide treatment to improve and restore function to the highest level of physical and mental well-being of the residents. Many times just improving a resident's attention span, through therapy, provides him with a higher quality of life. Sometimes occupational programs, such as bowling or paper and sewing crafts are offered through the activities department, as the two departments are closely related. If a nursing home has an occupational therapist, he should be certified by the American Occupational Therapy Association.

EXAMPLES OF THE
OCCUPATIONAL THERAPIST'S RESPONSIBILITIES

- Plans the department's therapy, its program, and activities
- Selects rehabilitative and therapeutic activities and exercises
- Reviews the occupational therapy policies and procedures
- Incorporates occupational therapy with the overall plan of care
- Provides guidance to staff in the ongoing care of the resident
- Discusses approaches to use in meeting the goals of occupational therapy
- Maintains the privacy of all residents in his care

Physical therapists use physical agents, such as walkers, parallel bars, slant boards, whirlpool, moist heat packs, massage, and exercise to restore residents' lost muscle tone and function. The physical therapist should be licensed by the State Board of Physical Therapist Examiners.

Mr. M., who had previously lived alone, fell and fractured a hip, underwent surgery, and was admitted to a nursing home. He became a candidate for physical therapy. Goals in his physical therapy are both short- and long-term. In Mr. M.'s case, the physician determined that the short-term goal would be to begin transfer-activity training (that is, teaching him to move back and forth from the wheelchair to the bed). The long-term goal would be to have Mr. M. return to independent living. Mr. M. attended physical therapy five times a week until the goals were met.

In addition to helping residents, a physical therapist teaches nursing home staff members the proper techniques of artificial limb application, exercise, and lifting.

EXAMPLES OF THE
PHYSICAL THERAPIST'S RESPONSIBILITIES

- Helps to maintain or restore the residents' physical functioning and prevent further deterioration
- Helps to develop plans to enhance the residents' sense of well-being
- Plans and develops the physical department's programs and activities
- Interprets physical therapy policies and procedures to personnel, residents, and family members when necessary
- Maintains the privacy of each resident and respects his wishes and requests

---

Licensed speech/language therapists help to treat and restore any type of cognitive (reading, writing, and math) deficit or swallowing impairment. These deficits and impairments may be the result of a stroke or of diseases such as multiple sclerosis or Lou Gehrig's disease.

Speech therapy is not used as often as physical therapy, so in most cases the speech therapist comes to the nursing home only on a consultant basis, but if the facility has a rehabilitation unit he may be employed at the facility on a full-time basis. The therapist will provide diagnostic screening and give recommendations for a speech therapy program; however, the attending physician must order the service.

EXAMPLES OF THE
SPEECH THERAPIST'S RESPONSIBILITIES

- Interviews residents and evaluates their need of therapy
- Recommends and develops a plan of therapy to meet the residents' needs
- Coordinates the services with the physician and nurses
- Records the residents' progress in his medical record and plan of care
- Recommends discharge and plans for continued care
- Maintains the privacy of each resident in his care

Dietitian

The dietary department is supervised by a registered dietitian (RD) who is a vital member of the nursing home.

Residents' health and outlook are affected by the food and atmosphere his department provides. A good dietitian will work to meet each resident's needs: if a resident has trouble chewing, the dietitian will provide soft food; if a resident needs to gain weight, the dietitian will plan extra snacks.

With the assistance of the occupational therapist, the dietitian provides special plate guards and additional implements to help residents feed themselves. By encouraging self-feeding, the dietitian helps promote independence and enhances residents' self-confidence.

The dietitian should make sure that meals and snacks are nutritional, pleasing in appearance, flavorful, served at proper temperatures, and cut up, ground, or pureed according to the individual residents' needs.

Occasionally families will ask, "What if Dad doesn't like a meal that's served?" If a resident refuses a meal, the dietitian should offer substitutions.

A choice of foods and a well-planned diet are both very important to residents in their own homes and must be provided in the long-term care facility. When a high quality of life is a priority, dietitians should be able to offer choices.

The dietary department is responsible for creating a pleasing environment in the main dining room. Some dietitians report an improvement in residents' appetites when the dining room is made restaurantlike, with linen tablecloths, fresh flowers on each table, newspapers, and coffee. In the nursing home where I worked, families were invited to join the residents for dinner or a buffet luncheon on holidays. Occasionally, dinner music was provided by a community organization.

EXAMPLES OF THE
DIETITIAN'S RESPONSIBILITIES

- Maintains a quiet, pleasant dining area by proper supervision of the dietary department
- Ensures balanced and attractively served meals
- Ensures that kitchen equipment is safe, clean, and modern
- Plans snacks for residents with diabetes as ordered by the physician
- Plans extra nourishments for residents according to the doctor's orders
- Participates in the residents' interdisciplinary plan of care
- Plans such therapeutic diets as diabetic, low-salt, and high- or low-calorie when needed

Housekeeping, Laundry, and Maintenance Workers

The housekeepers of a nursing home are responsible for the facility's general upkeep and appearance, and a careful look around will tell you how well they are doing their job. They are in charge of the residents' rooms as well as the common areas. They, too, should be careful to preserve residents' dignity. They should also know and practice techniques of careful handwashing so that they won't spread infection.

The laundry department is responsible for clothes and linens. Nursing homes will launder residents' personal clothing. However, since there is most often an extra charge for personal laundry, some families prefer to bring in a closed container for the soiled items and do the wash at home. Linens are either contracted out to a linen service or done at the facility.

The maintenance department is responsible for the general upkeep and repair of the building and all equipment. It should also keep the facility free of rodents and insects and instruct the nursing home staff in what to do in case of utility failure.

It is very difficult for a nursing home to find maintenance personnel who are qualified and who possess the traits necessary to work with older individuals in a caring and compassionate way while maintaining the residents' privacy. Yet a nursing home cannot function without maintenance workers, as they, like some of the other personnel, must be on call twenty-four hours a day.

EXAMPLES OF THE HOUSEKEEPERS', LAUNDRY WORKERS', AND MAINTENANCE WORKERS' RESPONSIBILITIES

- Maintain the safety of the nursing home
- Ensure that the staff is trained in emergency procedures in case of power failure
- Make frequent rounds of the nursing home to check the safe use of equipment
- Ensure adequate supplies of linens
- Treat the residents with respect and dignity
- Maintain the residents' privacy

The Interdisciplinary Patient Care Plan

The members of a nursing home's staff come together in interdepartmental, or interdisciplinary, meetings to plan and coordinate resident care. In these meetings, nurses, therapists, the activity director, the social worker, the dietitian, and other personnel all decide on realistic goals and approaches for each resident.

One interdepartmental team had to decide how best to help Mr. T., who was somewhat disoriented and had symptoms of arthritis, lack of bladder control, and constipation.

The team's first goal was to lessen the discomfort of his arthritis and prevent him from developing deformed joints. Under the doctor's direction, they provided medications as well as range of motion exercises. The team next discussed his loss of bladder control. To help Mr. T. become continent, the staff would take him to the bathroom every two hours while he was awake and offer him the bedpan during the night. A third goal, that of ensuring daily elimination, was handled by the dietitian, who would provide bran in Mr. T.'s morning cereal.

The social worker, noting Mr. T.'s family's lack of involvement with him, planned to try building a stronger relationship by holding meetings with the family members and involving them in discussion groups with other residents' families.

The activities director, who had noticed Mr. T.'s lack of contact with other people of his age, planned to involve him in a greater variety of group activities, including group sing-a-longs, story groups, and a discussion group. The director was aware that Mr. T. had been helpful in church organizations, so he would offer to bring him to weekly religious services.

A plan of care is written for each resident in the interdisciplinary meeting. This care plan becomes a permanent part of the resident's medical record and, at its best, ensures that the highest quality care will be provided for residents.

Having learned about the staff structure in a nursing home, their responsibilities, and how they coordinate their services, you can now begin to look at nursing homes in a more knowledgeable way, touring facilities, gathering information, and asking questions pertaining to quality of life and what it means to your loved one.

3

Choosing a Nursing Home

When you first decide to look for a nursing home, you may feel emotionally overwhelmed. It is normal to be depressed, anxious, angry, guilty, or scared at the thought of making such a big decision for yourself or a family member. Take comfort in the fact that your feelings are shared. Also, understand that if you follow the steps outlined in this chapter, your search for a nursing home will not be as difficult as you may imagine.

You can begin by gathering nursing home recommendations from people you respect, then narrow the possibilities and visit the nursing homes that seem most promising. During your visits, you will look for signs of high quality care and note problems. After the visits, compare the homes you've seen, considering price, quality, inspection reports, and location. Finally, with enough information, you will be ready to make a realistic choice.

The advice I give in this chapter is based on my years of work in nursing homes. While outside advisors may correctly tell you to check for adequate staffing, only a geriatric head nurse can tell you exactly what signs to look for when you visit a nursing home on a weekend evening. It is in the details of care that you find out about quality. Using the information here, you can make valuable observations about the quality of life a nursing home offers.

A word about choosing a nursing home: if you are seeking placement for a relative, try to involve her as much as possible in the decision-making. You can begin discussing changes in living accommodations long before a move is necessary. Remember, your relative will probably be as upset as you are at the thought of looking at nursing homes; my father considered nursing homes places of gloom and despair. While it may be difficult for you to bring up the subject, it is best to do so if you think a move to a nursing home might someday be necessary. If you begin the discussion early, you and your relative will have time to adjust, educate yourselves, and look for a good placement. Also, you may find that an early visit to a nursing home relieves you, since your worst fears will probably not be realized.

When you are ready to begin looking at nursing homes, let your relative know in a positive way. "You like going out for a drive. I'll treat you to lunch today and then we'll stop at the nursing home I saw on the way home. I'd like very much to show it to you and there are some people I'd like you to meet." Try not to make her feel that she's being pushed or coerced into the visit. If you let her decide which day is best for her, the timing of the trip becomes the decision to make rather than whether she wants to go.

It may happen that the moment you choose to broach the subject is not the best time for your relative to visit or meet people. But next week she may respond more positively to your suggestions. If you meet with an outright, emphatic, "No!" try again later.

Seeking Referrals

Before visiting nursing homes, get referrals from people in the field and from people who have been in situations similar to yours. You will find that you are not alone as you begin talking with your neighbors, friends, and relatives, many of whom have had experience with nursing homes. Also talk with geriatric counselors in hospitals. They can assist you in your selection. If your family member is presently a hospital patient, the hospital's social worker should be able to help. Read your local paper for articles about nursing homes and check the library for back articles on the subject.

Your family physician is another source of information. She may have patients in nursing homes and can tell you about the conditions in nearby facilities. She does not necessarily have to be the primary physician in charge of your relative. If she has been your physician, she should be willing to talk with you.

The state agencies on aging and the local long-term care ombudsman are additional sources of information. They cannot advise you on any one particular nursing home, but they will supply current information regarding nursing homes near you. If there are local advocacy groups or support groups for the aged and their families, they will also be good sources for recommendations.

Once you have a list of nursing homes, you will have to choose which to visit. If your list is short, you can see each one, but if the list is long, decide how many you can realistically look at and then select the ones that seem most likely to meet your needs.

Touring the Facility

There are two ways to look at nursing homes: on formal tours arranged through a nursing home's social worker and on informal, drop-in visits, which need not be prearranged. You can, and should, visit at various times throughout the day and weekends. You will especially want to visit during evening hours, as this is when a shortage of staff is most likely to occur. Administrative department heads are usually off on weekends and evenings, so you should try to see a nursing home at those times to get a realistic picture of how the staff operates without management supervision.

If your tour is self-conducted, it should begin outside the building. As you walk around, take particular notice of the general appearance and upkeep of the building. You can learn about the maintenance department this way. Maintenance is also in charge of lawns, porches, patios, and outdoor furniture. Are the patios used by the residents and are they equipped with outdoor furniture in good repair? Are there ramps at the doorways for wheelchairs?

Check the parking lot for good lighting and parking spaces. I have visited facilities that had both poor and inadequate parking conditions for employees and visitors. Will you have parking space available when visiting? Is the lighting adequate? Visiting during the evening hours will give you a good idea of how well the building is lit for easy and safe accessibility.

As you enter the building, look first at the common areas used by residents and their visitors. Most nursing homes have either one floor with several wings or several floors with two or three units on each floor and administrative offices on the main floor.

The majority of nursing homes have a central lobby and parlor where residents can socialize. You can check these areas for upkeep and maintenance. Are the areas neat, clean, and newly furnished or are the furnishings old and in need of cleaning and repair? Are the housekeepers busily trying to keep the areas clean and fresh or is there an objectionable, stale smell to the rooms? If residents are smoking in common areas, is there adequate ventilation? If a resident is a nonsmoker, she may find it very offensive to be exposed to smoking when she wants to socialize or visit with friends. Most nursing homes provide a special room for residents who smoke.

Handrails are installed on the walls of the corridors. Are these rails intact or are they loose and in need of maintenance? Floors must be repaired in a safe manner. Do you notice any holes in the floors that have been repaired with plastic tape? Are wall coverings in good repair or are they torn and patched poorly? Are linen carts covered neatly and do they appear clean?

Usually there is a main dining area for those who can walk or use their wheelchairs, although some homes have dining rooms in each nursing unit instead. It is an excellent idea to visit during mealtimes and take notice of these areas. Are they kept up and cleaned immediately after use? Are the floors free of food stains?

Next, go to the nursing units and check for sprinklers, smoke detectors, and fire extinguishers, which should be visible in hallways and nursing areas. All exits should be appropriately marked and lighted. Stairwells can be problem areas if doorways to these stairs are open to residents. Ask the nurses, as you tour, if the stairs are equipped with cameras or buzzers that inform the staff when someone has gone into a stairwell.

Pay particular attention to the noise level on the unit, since some facilities are known to be extremely noisy, disorganized, and chaotic. I have been in facilities with emergency buzzers (set up to clang much more loudly than is reasonable), intercom music and intercom messages (interspersed with the music), vacuum cleaners, floor buffers, blaring televisions, and patient room call-light bells all going at the same time! Is it any wonder that in state survey reports, inspectors can find "medication errors" or "errors in transcribing physicians' orders?" There is a strong possibility that errors are made because of undue noise and confusion on a unit. It is easy to detect noisy facilities, even if you are on a one-time tour. Fortunate are the residents and employees in facilities that provide "quiet rooms" for relaxation, meditation, or religious services.

Nurses' stations should be located in the center of each unit's halls with unobstructed views in all directions. Usually the corners of halls and entrances to sitting and dining areas have mirrors so that the staff can see around corners. Substandard nursing homes are not set up in this way, and nurses' stations often resemble small closets. Since no survey guidelines dictate the design of a nurse's desk area, there are many versions.

After leaving the nurse's station, you should look at the residents' rooms. A nurse may show you an unoccupied room but cannot infringe on an individual resident's privacy to show you an occupied one. While looking through an unoccupied room, check for grab bars and working sinks and toilets in the bathroom, screens on the windows, and one nightstand, bureau, and closet per person. Mirrors should be at a height appropriate to residents in wheelchairs. The beds should be made in all residents' rooms before the noon meal. Are the colors in the room bright and cheerful and does all the furniture match in color and design? As you walk by residents' rooms, notice if the call bells are within reach.

Nursing homes that offer a high quality of care make special accommodations for disoriented residents. I have seen some rooms of disoriented residents that have photographs of the resident on the door. This is especially helpful to a confused person, perhaps one with Alzheimer's disease, who has trouble finding his room. In one facility the activities director puts short autobiographies on each resident's door. This background information serves as the resident's introduction to the staff, other residents, and family members, and as a reorientation for a confused resident. Ask to see the unoccupied room of a disoriented resident. Does the room have orienting items around? Large numbers on clocks, drawers and beds labeled with the resident's name, and large numbered calendars are items to check for. Textures in fabrics and furnishings add warmth and a homelike appearance to a resident's room. Metal furnishings have the opposite effect. Soft color schemes are pleasing and tranquilizing to disoriented residents and to alert and oriented residents alike. Too many bright colors can cause overstimulation to already hyperactive residents. Does the facility have an enclosed outdoor area that disoriented residents can use?

Some facilities have installed the ultimate in comfort: a special room with an oversized whirlpool tub. This room may be referred to as the "spa" and requires a physician's order for use. There are beauty and barber shops in most facilities; if not, hair dressers and barbers should be available on call.

One of the main complaints that people visiting nursing homes have is about the odor. As you tour the nursing home, you should not notice an overwhelming, unpleasant smell in any part of the facility.

Talking to Residents and Staff

As you walk through the nursing home, take advantage of the chance to talk with people. You can gain valuable insight into the quality of life in the nursing home this way. When you see residents out of their rooms, take a few minutes to introduce yourself and perhaps explain that you are considering admission to the nursing home. Ask residents for their opinion of the facility. You may be fortunate enough to engage a resident's help in looking around. Notice if the residents are dressed neatly or if they are in their night-clothes in midmorning. Do they appear to be happy in their surroundings?

When residents don't want to talk about the nursing home, you may not be able to gain any insight from them and you will have to observe their behavior. For example, if they look unhappy, are very quiet and reluctant to talk to you, or appear apathetic about their surroundings, take another closer look at the facility! It may be that they are afraid of recrimination if they speak negatively of the facility. Don't doubt your own feelings about a nursing home! Chances are, what you are feeling is actually the truth about the facility.

If you are considering a particular nursing home, you must spend some time talking with the administrator. Is she receptive to your needs? Is she readily available when you ask for an appointment? Does she put you at ease and address your concerns? Remember, she will be in charge if your relative becomes a resident of this home.

It is also a good idea to talk with the nursing home social worker. She can arrange a more formal tour of the nursing home, pointing out areas you may have missed on an informal visit and directing you to the posted residents' bill of rights. She may also discuss topics such as which items to bring to the nursing home. She can provide a list of activities and general overall information concerning nursing home policies. If, after your tour and your meeting with her, you decide this nursing home is not the appropriate placement for your relative, the social worker can guide you to social service agencies in the community that can help you explore other living arrangements.

Aside from talking with the administrator and social worker, you will want to speak with the charge nurse and other personnel. Notice how they respond to your (and the residents') questions. Do staff members approach visitors in a calm manner and do they speak softly? If a nurse has time, you can ask her various questions about her unit and the residential floor.

Is there a refrigerator and hot plate on the unit for bedtime snacks? If not, ask what the staff does when a resident awakens and asks for some warm milk and cookies. Can alcoholic beverages be stored on the unit for your relative? Are extra supplies, such as toothbrushes, combs, and incontinence pads, kept on the units for easy accessibility? Some nursing homes keep supplies in a separate storage center away from the unit, accessible to only one person, usually a shift supervisor. If the delegated person is unavailable, an employee must wait until that person is able to answer a call. This can take anywhere from a few minutes to an hour or longer. Are ample supplies always available?

Notice the dress of the nursing staff. Employees should all look professional. It is the general opinion in health care that a resident feels more at home with a staff dressed in colors rather than in white uniforms. The white uniform shouts "hospital" and the modern nursing home is trying to separate itself from the hospital image. In some nursing homes you will find the nursing staff in colored tops and white pants. Sweat suit tops, dangling earrings, knee socks, and sandals or any other attire unbefitting to a professional nurse is not acceptable in a nursing home. Some charge nurses still wear white caps to distinguish them from the rest of the nursing staff. Others prefer only a large, easy-to-read name tag designating them as the charge nurse.

Evaluating Care

The most important contributor to a high quality of life in a nursing home is good interaction between residents and staff. Conversely, the biggest problems in a nursing home are caused by rude, thoughtless, careless, or overworked staff. When you visit a nursing home, you will have to observe staff members at work and evaluate the quality of care you see. The longer or more frequent your visits, the more information you will gather.

Listen to nursing assistants as they speak to residents. Do they stand directly in front of the person, speaking slowly and clearly so the resident can hear and see them? Do they occasionally touch the resident in a gentle, affectionate way while they talk? It is much more effective to talk to someone in a wheelchair when you stoop down so you are on eye level with them. Do you see the nurses standing, or stooping, close by the residents as they talk with them? Do they address their fellow workers in a quiet manner, or are they offensively loud in their approach? Listen to the way staff members react when a resident's behavior is inappropriate. Are they as kind at such times? It is always easy to be pleasant to someone who is alert and responds appropriately, but in a facility known for its high quality of care you will hear the staff respond just as pleasantly to the inappropriate requests of residents.

It is not difficult to detect a rude, uncaring, or defiant nurse or nursing assistant. She is the one who bumped into you as she came out of a resident's room. She didn't bother to stop and excuse herself but gave you a quizzical look and sneered as she waltzed by to the tune of a blaring radio in a resident's room. Mrs. Smith is calling out in distress to use the bedpan as Miss B., nursing assistant, is joking around with another worker in the hall. She may eventually go into Mrs. Smith's room, but she will roughly pick up the bedpan, put it on the bed, and leave the room without asking Mrs. Smith if she needs any help. Her attitude vaguely resembles that of a rebellious child. You can spot her by the rough way she acts toward the residents. She has no concern for the residents' emotional well-being, privacy and dignity, and she speaks to them in an unprofessional way. She is also likely to betray a resident's privacy and confidentiality.

Miss A. was one nurse who had no respect for her patients' privacy. One evening, she and I and a few other nurses were out to dinner near our nursing home. Before dinner was served, Miss A. began talking loudly about a resident whom she described as "a demanding and selfish patient who is always ringing the call bell." Later, when she turned around, she saw the resident's family sitting behind her. Confidentiality was furthermost from Miss A.'s mind.

One way to evaluate the care given by a charge nurse is to observe the activity levels of the residents in her charge. Do they sit for long periods with no one to talk to? Are they in the television room (or the hall) for great lengths of time with no diversion? Are they in the same area when you come for a repeat visit? If you find that residents are in different locations at various times and that the nurse is frequently talking and visiting with them, you can be sure that you have a person who is compassionate and motivated in caring for the emotional needs of the geriatric resident.

One measure of the care in a nursing home is the presence or absence of a certified medicine aide (CMA). It is almost impossible for a unit to function effectively without a CMA, or a licensed nurse whose sole responsibility it is to administer medications. I would be hesitant to admit a family member of mine to any nursing home without one. Yet I have worked in facilities without a "medicine nurse" on the unit. The administration of a nursing home should not minimize the need for such an important position.

As you evaluate the care given in a nursing home, pay particular attention to the way disoriented residents are handled. Many facilities are now beginning to make special provisions for residents with Alzheimer's disease. These patients tend to wander. They are confused, unaware of their surroundings, do not recognize familiar faces, and may be agitated or hostile. Specially trained personnel should provide the care these people require. Look, for example, in the television room, at the residents who are in specially designed geriatric chairs with locked trays. The residents in geriatric chairs are usually disoriented. Are their calls answered or do they go unheeded? In some nursing homes, the disoriented person can inadvertently be treated as though every sound she makes is an incoherent request. When Mrs. White says she's hungry twenty minutes after her tray is taken away, do you hear the nursing assistant tell her several different reasons why she can't possibly be hungry already? "You're so confused. You just *had* breakfast." "You don't know what you want." "Lunch will be here in three hours." "You didn't eat all your food when your tray was here, and now you want more." These are a few overheard responses to disoriented residents in substandard nursing homes.

Does the nursing staff show respect for the feelings expressed by the confused residents even though there is no answer to their requests? If Mrs. Brown cries that she misses her husband and the staff knows that he has been dead for many years, do you hear the nurses responding to her cries in a caring manner, "I know how you miss your husband, Mrs. Brown. I would miss mine, too, if he weren't around." Or do you hear an uncaring assistant telling Mrs. Brown that her husband is dead and has been for a long time and she won't be seeing him anymore? This is a response I heard as I was visiting my father at a nursing home.

Each resident's request should be treated as if made by an alert and oriented resident, and each individual resident should be treated with dignity at all times. Are these disoriented residents kept dry and clean by the staff and are they taken to the toilet at regular intervals, especially after meals?

Consider also how disoriented residents are treated at mealtime. They should have the opportunity to use the common dining areas. A disoriented person does not have to be seated next to alert and oriented residents, especially if she must be fed. Such seating could be very upsetting to oriented residents as well as to the confused resident. The oriented individual might be alarmed by what could lie ahead for her in the future. Disruptive residents should be taken to another area of the dining room.

Mealtime in general, and the evening meal in particular, is a good time to visit a nursing home and observe the quality of care. Evening meals are the most difficult time of day. This is the moment when many residents who have been out of bed all day are becoming tired and more easily agitated. Do you notice that the staff is caring and gentle in their approach to the resident? Do they stop and ask the residents if they are still hungry or thirsty, need to go to the bathroom, or would like to take a bath and go to bed early? Do they clean up the dining and television rooms as they go along? Do they help all the residents who need and ask for help? Are the dietary personnel respectful to the residents? Do they respond promptly to requests? Do you hear residents asking for substitute choices, and are other foods made available to them? After the residents are taken back to the nursing unit, is the main dining area attended to and cleaned up by the housekeeping department?

After you have observed the care given by nurses and assistants, look at the activities department. In my opinion, this department, next to nursing, is the most important in the facility. What activities occupy a resident's interests and keep her functioning at her optimal levels mentally, emotionally, and physically? What programs are available to help motivate her? Can she be encouraged to help others? The director of the activity department asks herself these questions about each resident and uses the answers to plan resident programs.

The old as well as the young need interaction and, at times, require external motivation. An individual cannot always be self-motivated. Occasionally a resident needs the stimulation of other people and activities to keep her mentally active and involved in something that she considers worthwhile. Even the individual who prefers to be alone needs an occasional get-together. The activities director must find a way to appeal to all types of residents. Mental stagnation and loneliness can occur in people who are left to their own devices for long periods. In the same way that exercise deters the development of physical problems, meaningful activities can help ward off symptoms of mental suffering.

Activities provided in a nursing home must be suited to the older person without demeaning her capabilities and mentality. The goal of most activities is to provide a resident with a meaningful way to help herself while helping others. If she can maintain her dignity and sense of self-worth, her feelings of loneliness, self-involvement, depression, and frustration will be greatly diminished.

Some nursing homes have better activities than others. Ask for a calendar that lists activities for that month. The best nursing homes will have a wide range of programs: hobby and craft groups, serious and light-hearted discussion groups; competitive activities for those who enjoy them; and extensive musical programs. Social outings in the community should be an integral part of the activity program. Since religion provides a strong support system for many of the elderly, the activities department should provide religious services and programs and invite clergy to visit with residents.

Included in all the best nursing homes is a regularly scheduled physical exercise program. A sign posted in a Pennsylvania nursing home's activity room tells us that, "You can't turn back the clock, but you can sure wind it up again." Daily exercise helps the long-term care resident strengthen her muscles, feel more energetic, and raise her self-esteem. Exercise groups also provide social interaction with others. In some facilities the staff is encouraged to join in the exercise and the fun.

Ask the activities director how she handles the difficult issue of mixing oriented and disoriented residents in the same programs. There may be activities not suited to some disoriented people, and for these residents, programs are arranged on a one-to-one basis. However, the fact that an individual is noisy and disruptive one day should not preclude her attendance at a program another day. There can be definite physical reasons for agitation and nervousness; it may require several days of monitoring by the staff to determine the cause. Once the problem has been resolved, the resident should again be brought into the group and invited to participate. In this way, the director can provide an ongoing, active program for all residents, tailored to their needs.

There are good reasons for activities directors to work at mixing oriented and disoriented residents. Not only does the mixed group offer a disoriented person the opportunity for increased mental remotivation and a more meaningful existence, it also allows an alert resident to give of herself. In so doing, she may feel not just a sense of helping her fellow resident but also an inner gratitude that she is still in control of her faculties. Sometimes a great closeness, like that between a parent and child, grows between the giver and the receiver. However, it is not realistic to expect that mixed groups will always work. It is important for you to observe and ask about homogenous grouping of residents in the nursing home.

One of the best ways to learn about all aspects of a nursing home's care is to volunteer to work in the activities department. By doing this, you become aware of the inner workings of a nursing home and can better decide if a particular facility will meet your relative's needs.

As you evaluate the quality of care a nursing home provides, you will realize that many intangibles are involved. No agency can evaluate the human kindness and compassion demonstrated by dedicated employees; no standard mandates that someone will have a shoulder to cry on or a loving hand to hold; no grading system can be devised for a nursing assistant who sits with a dying resident on her day off or visits on a holiday or a resident's birthday. Regulations do not govern the remotivation of a lonely, elderly widow. Can anyone begin to document the hours a caring social worker spends with a resident? No surveyor is present the day a nursing assistant, on her lunch hour, plants flowers around the front entry of a nursing home for all to enjoy.

Such warm and happy moments do exist in nursing homes, but no governing agency inspects a home for these intangibles. During your nursing home visits, be sure to look and see if there are staff members who give more than is expected, who go the extra mile.

Comparing Nursing Homes

I once took a prospective resident's family on a brief tour of two nursing homes. After they had completed the first tour, I asked for their impressions of the facility. I was very interested in their opinions, since they had not been in a nursing home before. Their response was that nobody in the nursing home looked happy, including the staff. They said the surroundings appeared gloomy and drab, uninteresting, unstimulating, and lacking in color. The entire atmosphere, they said, was depressing. I then took them on a tour of another facility. Their response changed: "Now that we have seen another nursing home, we can speak comparatively. This home was much brighter in its lighting and the colors were more cheerful and refreshing. The residents appeared happy. The employees talked to us as we walked through and even asked if they could be of help. Many activities were taking place and for those who were not engaged in activities, there were volunteers who would read to them on the patio. Also, in the first nursing home we saw residents being pulled around in shower chairs. They weren't being pushed like you would push someone in a wheelchair, but pulled backwards!" I explained that these were just a few factors to consider when looking at nursing homes.

A family should consider a checklist to take along with them when touring a facility. Comparison shopping is essential when considering nursing home placement. Before making a choice, you will have to consider some important factors—quality of life, cost, and location—and weigh the pluses and minuses of each potential placement.

As a result of your nursing home visits and your review of inspection reports, you will have evaluated the quality of care offered by each institution. Perhaps you found one nursing home that offered everything you wanted; more likely, you saw homes that were less than perfect but still acceptable. Unfortunately, there is often a shortage of space at the best nursing homes and there might be a waiting list at the one you prefer. If you are not pressed for time, you can put your name on the list, but if you need a quick placement, you will have to settle for a second or third choice.

The deciding factor for most families in choosing a nursing home is cost. (Costs and methods of payment are discussed in detail in the next chapter.) At each facility you visit, ask about fees and extra charges and find out if Medicare and Medicaid payments are accepted. Once you know what nursing home care will cost, you can decide which homes are affordable, based on your ability to pay.

FINANCIAL QUESTIONS TO ASK OF A NURSING HOME

- What are the set fees and what services do they cover?
- Are there extra charges?
- If a resident leaves the home, does she receive a refund?
- Does the home accept Medicare and Medicaid patients?
- How are payments to be made?
- What happens if the resident runs out of private funds?
- How often does the nursing home bill increase?
- Does private insurance pay any of the bill?
- Are the charges higher on your unit for a resident with Alzheimer's disease?

Don't make any decision about a nursing home until you understand all the financial obligations and arrangements involved. Keep asking questions of the social workers, administrators, and admissions directors, and consult a lawyer about contracts and legalities. A nursing home should always give you time to clear up your uncertainties before asking you to sign any papers. Nursing homes have admissions contracts. Ask for one to take with you. Study it before signing.

You may find that the nursing home you would like to choose for its quality of life charges a fee that is too high for you or your family member to pay. In such a case, you will have to compromise and pick the best possible affordable placement.

The last important factor to consider when choosing a nursing home is its location. The best way to ensure good care for your relative once she becomes a resident is to visit often and act as an advocate, and it is hard to do this if you are far from the nursing home. When weighing care and cost, keep in mind that your frequent presence can contribute greatly to your relative's quality of life.

There are many important facts to consider when touring nursing homes. I want to stress again the most important of all—the residents. They are the ones, by both communication and behavior, who can tell you about their quality of life, likes and dislikes, and needs.

In Chapter 4, you will learn how to help pay for nursing home care, the details of the Medicare and Medicaid programs, and what happens when Medicare is denied.

4

Arranging for Payments

The cost of nursing home care is staggering; for most Americans it represents an enormous financial burden. Only those who can pay up to $3,000 or so per month, and the very poor, whose expenses are paid by Medicaid, escape the hardship of monthly bills. If you have decided that a nursing home stay is necessary for your relative, you must deal with the problem of financing the care. It is not enough to plan, as I have seen some families do, for the first few months and then hope that some additional financing will come along. You should take a realistic look at your expenses and sources of funds, and learn as much as possible about the major means of financing care. A side benefit of educating yourself is that you will be less likely to fall prey to those unscrupulous nursing homes and insurance companies that take financial advantage of the elderly.

There are a number of ways to pay for nursing home care: through Medicare, Medicaid, the Veterans Administration, private sources such as personal assets, and insurance. You may depend solely on one method or may combine methods of payment. However, you should know that not all nursing homes are certified to accept Medicare and Medicaid payments, and not all homes take residents covered under the Veterans Administration. You will find quite a few homes that accept only residents who pay for their care privately.

Here is a brief explanation of the main payment methods. Medicare is the government program for which all entitled citizens over age sixty-five qualify,. free of charge. The program requires that care be provided by a skilled nursing home. Unlike Medicare, Medicaid is *not* available to everyone; a person must qualify financially and medically to become eligible for this program for the indigent. The

Veterans Administration funding, available to those who are eligible, pays for several months of nursing home care for a person admitted from a VA hospital.

This chapter will tell you in detail about private funding, Medicare, and Medicaid, and will describe the problems people face in trying to pay for care. I have seen some creative solutions to financing, but I have also seen some sad cases.

After Mrs. M.'s husband died, I asked her how she had managed, on her own, to pay for his extensive long-term care at a nursing home. Years before, when my father had been ill, my husband and I had been able to pay for his nursing home care for only a short time. An extended stay at the facility would have completely depleted our savings.

Mrs. M.'s husband had had a stroke and had been admitted to a nursing home. Mrs. M. had savings accounts that she planned on using to pay for her husband's care. After four years of payments, her savings were depleted. She didn't know how she could continue paying privately for his care, so she began considering the state's Medicaid program. However, to fulfill Medicaid eligibility requirements she would have had to first sell her home and use the proceeds to pay for her husband's care. Just thinking about giving up the home that she and her husband had built and filled with such happy memories caused Mrs. M. a great deal of emotional pain. She couldn't do this to her husband! She would think of some other way to continue his care at the nursing home but she would not sell their home. She sold her oil paintings and antique jewelry and paid for an additional three months' care. After that, she was again faced with the financial worry of continued nursing home payments and the possibility that she would have to apply for Medicaid. She sought professional advice and was reminded of her husband's stocks and bonds and the income they would bring if she liquidated them, which she eventually did.

Her mental and physical health declining, Mrs. M. one day received a call from the nursing home saying that her husband needed hospitalization for another stroke. After three weeks in the hospital, Mr. M. was readmitted to the nursing home but this admission was paid for by

*Medicare. After ten days, Mrs. M. received a call saying
that her husband had passed away. She was left a
widow with few resources for her own support. What a
sad way to end a couple's life.*

Not everyone has stocks, bonds, jewelry, and oil paintings
to relinquish in the hope of sustaining nursing home care
for a loved one, nor is everyone blessed with enough
physical and mental stamina to take the rigors of financial
and medical worries. Fortunately, there is now recognition
of the hardship of paying for nursing home care. Recently
enacted legislation has changed Medicaid requirements to
help protect spouses from impoverishment and financial
ruin if a nursing home becomes necessary. Also, some
private insurance companies are beginning to offer limited
nursing home coverage for the elderly, but this amount is
only about 1 percent of the total cost of the nursing home.

Since the news about Medicare, Medicaid, private funding,
and payments changes constantly, you should keep
informed by reading news accounts and contacting advocacy
groups such as the National Citizens Coalition, the American
Association of Retired People (AARP), and the Alzheimer's
Disease and Related Disorders Association (ADRDA). (See
Appendix D.) You can also get information about funding
from your state and local social service agencies, your
senators, and your congressional representatives. To arrange
personal funding, you might consider talking to financial
planners, insurance agents, or bank loan officers. And
through local and national community action organizations,
you can work to help ease the burden of heavy nursing
home costs. Making high quality nursing home care affordable for all who need it should be a national goal.

Using Private Sources

The Older Women's League reports the average nursing
home cost to be $25,000 annually, with facilities in the
northeast being the most expensive. If a nursing home
resident pays privately, the money for his care comes from
his own resources or from those of his family. Some
residents are able to finance their stay through savings, but
many are forced to sell off their assets.

If your relative will be using private sources for payment,
you will want to be particularly thorough when looking at

nursing home costs. It is not enough to consider monthly rates when comparing nursing homes. Rates are variable, depending on the kind of accommodation (single or double room), the supplies and services needed, the "extras" available, and the location. For example, let's consider two facilities, compare their monthly rates, and look at the services that are included.

Nursing Home AB

$3,000.00 per month
+   40.00 laundry
+   15.00 ironing
Monthly fee includes: room, board, spoon-feeding, incontinence pads, and items such as tissues, powder, and body lotion.

Nursing Home CD

$2,300.00 per month
+   3.00 per day incontinence care
+   4.00 per day spoon-feeding
+   15.00 one dozen incontinence pads
+   2.00 tissue
+   30.00 laundry/ironing
Monthly fee includes: room and board.

At Nursing Home AB, a total monthly bill including laundry provisions is $3,055 and includes care that a resident may not currently need. At Nursing Home CD, while the monthly bill is lower, $2,354 (including laundry charges), the amount charged is based on the care received. If a time comes when the resident needs spoon-feeding every day plus incontinence care and pads, he might receive a monthly bill much higher than $3,055. Note: In a metropolitan area the above two nursing homes could be $1,000 a month higher.

Here is something else to consider when weighing the costs of nursing homes: many of the supplies and services that you would assume are paid for under the monthly bill, are not. Almost all homes will charge your relative for enema supplies, catheters, rubber gloves for treatment, bandages, syringes for injections and tube feedings, hand and skin lotions, and urine testing materials. Doctor, pharmacy, and surgical supply company charges are not included in the basic nursing home bill. If you rent or buy a walker, wheelchair, geriatric chair, or cane, this is an additional cost. Physical and speech therapies are additional costs.

Occasionally, a family using private funds can save money on needed supplies by looking through classified ads in the newspaper for used items. The various resource centers listed in Appendix D may provide some of the needed items free of charge. When my father was living with me I obtained dressings and supplies through the American Cancer Society.

If you or your relative is planning to finance nursing home care privately, make sure the nursing homes you are considering spell out exactly what your true costs will be. Only with complete information can you make realistic plans for payment.

Medicare

Medicare is federal health insurance offering hospital coverage, optional doctors' fee coverage, limited home health care and nursing home care coverage.

WHO IS ELIGIBLE FOR MEDICARE?

- People sixty-five or older who are entitled to social security benefits
- People under sixty-five who are disabled
- People insured, under Social Security or by the Railroad Retirement Board, who need kidney dialysis or a kidney transplant
- People employed by the federal government for a specific period who need kidney dialysis or a kidney transplant

---

The Health Care and Financing Administration administers the Medicare program, but your relative's health insurance card will be issued by the Social Security Administration. The Railroad Retirement Board issues cards for the railroad's retirement beneficiaries. The Medicare card will identify your relative by name, sex, health insurance claim number, and the date of his entitlement to the insurance plan. The Social Security Administration is responsible for hearings and appeals on individuals' rights to Medicare benefits.

Medicare regulations change often, so use the information in this chapter as a general guide and get specifics about your relative's case from your hospital social worker, nursing home admissions counselor, or local social services office.

Medicare consists of two parts. Part A covers hospitalization and, under strict guidelines, a period of recuperation at home or in a skilled nursing home. The nursing home must be licensed as skilled and certified to receive Medicare funds. Part A is free but does have a deductible ($592 in 1990 and increased on January 1 of each year) that your relative will have to pay before he receives hospital benefits. Medicare Part B is optional insurance that covers medical and doctors' bills not already covered under Part A. Again, there are strict guidelines governing payments and a monthly premium ($28.60 in 1990 and increased each year), after meeting a $75 deductible.

Medicare Part A

Here is how Part A works. If your relative has been hospitalized for three or more consecutive days, a doctor certifies the need for skilled nursing services, your relative enters a *skilled*, Medicare certified nursing home within thirty days, and meets other criteria for coverage, Medicare Part A might pay full coverage for his care in a nursing facility for the first twenty days. If it is determined that he needs continued skilled services, Medicare Part A will continue to pay all but $74.00 a day (in 1990) for up to eighty more days. If your relative is a privately paying resident, he has to pay the $74.00.

Upon admission to the nursing home, your relative's care and medical chart is reviewed by a group made up of nurses and doctors. This group is called a utilization review committee and will periodically review his progress. The committee looks for specific criteria to be met before Medicare Part A will pay, or continue to pay, for his skilled nursing home care.

The 100 days of nursing home coverage is called a benefit period and to be eligible for a new benefit period, covered by Medicare Part A in a nursing home, your relative would have to be discharged from a skilled level of care for a period of sixty days and then be again admitted to a hospital for a minimum of three days. If, on readmission to a skilled facility, his care meets the criteria specified by Medicare, a new benefit period would begin.

Who determines how long your relative's bill will be covered by Medicare Part A? The review committee who approved Medicare Part A when he was admitted to the nursing home makes the initial determination and continues to monitor his case at regular intervals. As soon as your relative's care becomes routine, they will suggest discontinuing Medicare Part A coverage.

When Medicare Part A will no longer pay for the nursing home stay, it is called a "denial" of coverage. This denial of coverage can result from the review committee's suggestion of discontinuing Medicare Part A or by his having received the maximum 100-day Medicare Part A coverage for the year.

When Medicare Part A is denied, federal guidelines mandate that several people be notified by mail: the attending physician, the facility administrator, the resident, and/or whoever is responsible for his bills. This notification is called a denial letter and states why a continued stay at the nursing home does not qualify for additional payment by Medicare.

On first appearance, the denial letter can represent a real threat. The attending physician and/or the family and the resident, if unfamiliar with Medicare guidelines, may think the resident has to leave the facility immediately. However, a denial letter does not mean a resident is considered able to care for himself or that he has to leave the nursing home. The letter simply says that skilled services are no longer necessary and that methods of payment other than Medicare must be used for nursing home care. The letter may look like the example below.

SAMPLE DENIAL LETTER

To _____ Beneficiary _____   _____ Issued date _____

Medicare regulations require notification that the named beneficiary no longer meets the Medicare program requirements and therefore, beginning on (date)_____,
you are responsible for payment of your continued stay. The last date services furnished may be covered under Medicare (Part A or B) is (date) _____ .

The reason for this determination is that _____.

THIS DENIAL DOES NOT MEAN YOU MUST LEAVE THE NURSING HOME. EITHER THE MEDICAID PROGRAM OR YOU WILL BE RESPONSIBLE FOR THE SERVICES.

AN APPEAL OF THIS DECISION CAN BE MADE THROUGH THE LOCAL SOCIAL SECURITY OFFICE. TAKE THIS LETTER WITH YOU.

A denial of Medicare Part A might happen as soon as a resident enters a nursing home or anytime afterwards. Although Medicare Part A has been denied, if, within thirty days, he again needs skilled services, Medicare Part A will pay. Because of the potential for Medicare denials, admissions directors are very concerned about how prospective and current residents plan to pay for care.

Mr. A, for example, is a resident who did not require a skilled nursing home.

Mr. A., a long-time nursing home resident, fell and fractured his hip. He was able to walk around at the hospital after having surgery, and returned to the nursing home, where he received physical therapy five times a week. The committee that reviewed his case on admission denied him Medicare benefits because his physical therapy did not require the services of a skilled therapist. Rather, his therapy could be given by a nursing assistant or companion and therefore Medicare Part A would not pay for the skilled nursing home stay.

Even though the hospital staff told Mr. A that his care would be paid for by Medicare in the nursing home, this was not the case. The hospital staff does not always know what Medicare Part A will cover in the nursing home. Only the utilization committee can determine if Medicare Part A might pay for the nursing home. Some residents and families have been misinformed by well-meaning hospital staff, and for that reason admissions directors at nursing homes are very quick to ask about the payment source.

EXAMPLES OF SERVICES NOT COVERED BY MEDICARE PART A

- Giving eye drops
- General care of casts and braces
- General care of artificial limbs
- Routine assistance with a colostomy
- Routine assistance with daily activities and incontinence care
- Skilled rehabilitation services done only once or twice a week

---

MEDICARE PART A MIGHT COVER THESE SERVICES

- Skilled physical therapy (if criteria is met)
- Frequent adjustments of medication, based on laboratory results
- Dressing changes that must be done by a nurse
- Suctioning of residents' airways to prevent choking
- Teaching residents to give themselves injections or treatments
- Skilled observation and monitoring of terminally ill residents
- Daily insulin injections

Many families don't realize that they may jeopardize their relative's Medicare coverage by taking him out of the facility for overnight visits. The Medicare program requires that a resident needing a skilled nursing facility for his care receive the care on a twenty-four hour a day basis. Always check with the charge nurse before taking your relative out of the facility.

Medicare Part B

Medicare Part B, called supplementary insurance, is coverage for the medical and doctors' bills not covered by Part A and is optional. Your relative may be eligible for Part B insurance even if he does not have Part A of Medicare coverage. When an annual deductible of $75 is met, Part B will pay 80 percent of your relative's *approved* physicians' bills, supplies, and services and the other 20 percent (copayment) is paid by him. The premium for Medicare Part B was $28.60 in 1990 and is increased each year.

MEDICARE PART B MIGHT COVER THESE SERVICES

- Outpatient physical and speech therapy
- Medical and laboratory tests
- Dressings, splints and casts
- Braces, artificial limbs and repairs to these devices
- Ambulance services (when necessary)

All the services billed under Part B must be medically necessary and are subject to medical review. It helps to have a physician's order for necessary medical equipment or services.

MEDICARE PART B WILL NOT COVER
• Routine foot care • Eye and hearing examinations • Immunizations (but certain influenza vaccines are covered)

Medicare is a complex and sometimes overwhelming system. In 1986, a federally mandated Outreach Program was started to answer Medicare beneficiaries' questions, primarily ones related to the reconsideration and appeal processes. The program can help you understand Medicare and let you know of your rights and responsibilities. Each state has its own information center. You can contact the Health Care and Financing Administration (see Appendix D) for information on the Outreach Program.

You can also get additional information on Medicare program benefits and allowable expenses by writing to your local Consumer Affairs Office and asking for a copy of the "Medicare Supplement Insurance Guide." In addition, you can request Publication #05-10043 from the Social Security office or write to the Health Care Financing Administration (see Appendix D) for handbook #10050. Because there are so many questions on the new Medicare guidelines, a hotline number has been set up. Dial 1-800-888-1998 for immediate response to your questions.

Since Medicare does not cover all medical costs, it is suggested that people supplement Medicare coverage with private insurance coverage. These supplementary plans are called "Medigap" plans. Unscrupulous companies have used various scare tactics to enroll the elderly in policies that duplicated Medicare. Make an appointment to talk with someone in your local Office of Consumer Affairs or Social Security Office. They can provide you or your relative with pamphlets and information and discuss various options with you.

Medicaid

If your relative is unable to pay privately and is limited in financial resources, he may be eligible for Medicaid, which is insurance for the indigent. Both state and federal monies fund Medicaid, with most funding to nursing homes provided through Title XIX of the Social Security Act. State agencies determine whether a facility qualifies for Medicaid funding. The Health Care and Financing Administration relies on inspection surveys to ensure that high-quality care is being provided by these nursing homes in order for them to receive Medicaid funding. The availability of Medicaid funds differs from state to state, depending on per capita income, and each state governs its welfare program differently.

Up until the new Medicaid impoverishment protection of 1988, people who needed Medicaid often found that they were ineligible because of their state's requirements. Even a person with limited income did not always meet the financial requirements because of savings, investments, property, or insurance. In some states, the net worth of a family was taken into consideration when a person applied for Medicaid. In some states a person couldn't qualify for Medicaid until most of his assets had been sold. This is called "spending down." In such a case, only personal items such as clothes, furniture, and a limited amount of money for burial expenses could be kept.

The following story is an example of the sad situations which used to come about prior to spousal impoverishment protection:

Mr. P., a 30-year-old husband and the sole financial provider for his wife and twelve-year-old child, was hospitalized with multiple sclerosis. The physician told Mrs. P. that her husband would never work again and that his medical bills would become astronomical. Furthermore, he explained, it would not be possible to provide Mr. P.'s care at home. He would need nursing home supervision. Mrs. P. had not worked since her marriage and was now responsible for the care of both her child and her disabled husband. Her husband was to be discharged from the hospital but she had no money to pay privately for a nursing home, so she applied for Medicaid for him. However, she was then faced with the prospect of going on welfare, since, if she went to work, her salary would disqualify her husband from the Medicaid program. Mrs. P.'s solution to this dilemma was to get a divorce so that she and her child could stay off welfare and her husband (now her former husband) could receive nursing home care paid for by the state.

Even if your relative enters a nursing home as a privately paying resident, he may eventually find it necessary to apply for Medicaid. Most people have not saved enough to pay privately for a lengthy nursing home stay. Why is it that such an expensive and often necessary living arrangement (with one out of every four elderly people eventually needing nursing home care) is not saved for in the same manner as a vacation or retirement plan? The answer is that nursing homes are not a topic for the young or middle aged during good health and prosperity. The financial focus during these years is directed toward immediate needs: food, clothing, shelter, vacations, the children's college education, and, if possible, investments.

A neighbor recently told me that her parents were paying for their nursing home room at the rate of $6500 a month! In just a few months they would spend their lifetime savings on a nursing home room and have to apply for Medicaid. It is estimated that the average couple's savings is depleted after about a year's stay in a nursing home.

During our discussion of nursing homes' costs, my friend said, "My parents had always said they would rather die than spend their remaining days paying for a nursing home." I, too, have heard this said, especially by young people. However, when faced with a debilitating illness, some people reverse their opinions and reassess their feelings toward nursing homes. Quality of life issues may be different at such a time than when they were younger and enjoying good health. Sustaining life becomes the most important issue. A nursing home is then viewed as a respite, a hope, and a place to live their remaining days in dignity and comfort.

And what happens when your money has been depleted? Will you qualify for the Medicaid program? The amount your relative must "spend down" to qualify financially for Medicaid depends on state regulations. Anything over this amount will make him ineligible for Medicaid. The time required to complete the necessary Medicaid paperwork is so long and the number of applications received by social service offices is so great that it could take months before your relative is granted Medicaid funding.

You may wonder what happens to the resident who was paying privately for his care at the nursing home, used up all his money, and now has been approved by the Medicaid program both financially and medically. Does he have to find another nursing home or can he stay where he is since he is satisfied with his care? If the nursing home is certified by the Medicaid program, he can stay where he is but not all homes choose to participate in Medicaid. If you think your relative may eventually need the Medicaid program, make this one of your questions before considering the nursing home.

Whether your relative has been living at home or in a nursing home, he must, in order to be eligible for Medicaid, not only qualify financially, but also medically as certified by a physician. The physician will document your relative's necessary level of care and a state medical review agent will either approve or deny medical eligibility for the state's Medicaid program based on his medical needs.

If your family member is accepted by Medicaid, his nursing home bill is paid for by the government, which pays the difference between the amount the nursing home charges and his contribution (by way of Social Security checks or other monthly incomes). Your relative will be allowed to keep only a small amount for personal spending from his monthly incomes. One reason that holidays at nursing homes are special times is that different community organizations donate many little gifts, such as soaps, perfumes, candy, or cookies, which mean so much to those who cannot afford to buy these items during the year.

If your relative is receiving funding from the Medicaid program, his case will be reviewed periodically by an agent contracted by the state. Your relative may be denied a continued stay at a nursing home based on his medical needs. If he is denied a continued stay, he, the nursing home, and his physician will receive a denial letter including instructions on how to appeal the decision.

Fraudulent Charges

You must stay on top of your relative's financial situation, since there are nursing homes that take advantage of residents. Some facilities wrongfully continue an individual's private paying status after he has become eligible for Medicaid. Other nursing homes have solicited monetary contributions as a condition of admission to or a continued stay at the nursing home.

One unsuspecting prospective resident was told he could have a room at the nursing home if he signed over all his life insurance policies, sold his car and home, and also gave his jewelry and antiques to the nursing home owner. He was assured he'd be cared for as long as he needed. The home was not licensed or certified to receive Medicare or Medicaid funding, so the owner was not subject to the strict survey and auditing of his books which would normally protect this resident.

At hearings before the Special Committee on Aging in 1984 and 1985, some admissions directors testified that they had been instructed by the owner/administrator of a nursing home to maintain separate waiting lists—one for privately paying residents and one for residents covered by Medicaid—and to fill beds with the privately paying people first. According to the committee's report, one home moved a resident from one area of the facility to a less desirable one on the day that the resident changed from being privately paying to using Medicaid.

Perhaps one reason for fraudulent charges and discrimination is the problem of cost reimbursement to nursing homes. Nursing home administrators say that neither the Medicaid nor the Medicare programs reimburse for all the services a nursing home provides its residents. One administrator testified before the Special Committee on Aging that since there is a Medicare ceiling reimbursement rate based on a nursing home's cost history, and since facilities are now admitting patients needing more skilled services, the cost of care is rising more rapidly than reimbursement levels.

Congress has authorized the states to set their own reimbursement rate for Medicaid funding to nursing homes, but requires that it be sufficient. The facilities must not compromise high-quality nursing care to meet the costs of operating with state funds.

In this chapter we have discussed the methods of payment that might be used for nursing home care. We have also discussed the fraudulent methods that have been used by owners and administrators of nursing homes more concerned with money than with the quality of life of its residents. What all this means to you is that you and your relative must be diligent about monitoring costs, checking on nursing home billing procedures, and asking questions and then asking again, if you are not sure of the answers.

You should not be intimidated by an administrator when asking questions about costs and about Medicare and Medicaid information. Seeking legal advice is sound practice where finances are concerned. Finances are a confusing and unpleasant part of care for the elderly, but if you pay attention to costs and money, you will help maintain the best affordable quality of life for yourself or your relative.

5

Moving to a Nursing Home

Feelings about the Change

One of the hardest decisions I have ever had to make was moving my father into a nursing home. To him, the move meant the loss of close and joyful family relationships. He was saddened at the prospect of leaving his home and losing his freedom and independence. And he worried about which of his friends would want to visit him in a nursing home. He agreed that a nursing home was necessary but nevertheless he was emotionally upset and distraught. He knew that I could no longer care for him at home and that no other living arrangement had worked out, yet it seemed there had to be another answer. When the time comes that you have to make this decision, most likely you too will feel the overwhelming sense of despair and depression.

Everyone involved in the process of admission to a nursing home is likely to be upset. This is a natural feeling. It is not unusual for an elderly person, afraid of the coming move, to try to make her family feel guilty. She may say, "How could you do this to me?" "No, I don't want to go." "You're just trying to get rid of me so you can travel." "You want to use up all my money behind my back." "You'll sell all my furniture and then I can never come home." At such a difficult time, you will feel a wide range of emotions, some of which you may have trouble acknowledging. Yet your guilt, anger, and frustration, or relief are all normal emotions, shared by others in similar situations.

Because of your relative's feelings, and your own, you may be anticipating a traumatic move to the nursing home. Yet there are a number of steps you can take to lessen everyone's tension and help make admission go smoothly.

First, involve your relative as much as possible in

decisions related to the move. Decisions should not all be made for her or she will feel resentment and hostility. Begin by talking to her about this crossroad in her life. Explain that friends and relatives will be there to help and to share her feelings. Her needs should not be ignored and she must not feel alone.

Honesty is not just the best policy, but the only policy to follow with your relative, and not just before admission day but at all times. Perhaps the most damaging thing you can do is to suggest that she will soon be taken home. While that may be everyone's ultimate goal, it is nearly impossible to predict when—if ever—such a move will be made. This thought, sometimes planted with the best of intentions or to alleviate the guilt a family member feels on admission day, soon comes to dominate all others in the resident's mind: not because the nursing home is a bad place, but because everyone naturally wants to be in their own home.

My father was worried that the move to the nursing home would shut off the possibility of going home. Reassurance was needed to remind him of our love and that I wouldn't be selling his furniture or getting rid of his personal belongings. I told him, "I promise I will leave everything as it is for now." Another of his fears was that of having to give up driving his car. His car represented the freedom to come and go when and if he pleased. Since he was not incompetent, he continued to drive even after he went to the nursing home. Other people are more concerned about their money, finances, and mail. They may feel that you will spend all their money. You may try telling your relative, "No, we won't spend your money. You can have access to it, to your valuables and jewelry, and to your private income. Your mail will come directly to you if that's what you want." Your relative will probably be relieved to hear this and may ask that you receive her mail at home and help her with her accounts when you visit with her.

Preparations for admission to a nursing home should always be conducted at a slow, unhurried pace. This will help you and your relative put as much thought and love into this relocation as you put into the move to any new home. Take time to talk about old days and memories and allow time for extra hugs and touching. It's also important to allow sufficient time to discuss the fears and concerns that are a natural part of entering a long-term care facility. Moving into a nursing home can mean a new life for your relative, freedom from the worries that literally cripple many of our elderly. Like any big change, it takes time to adjust to the situation.

Not all admissions to a nursing home can be relaxed, orderly, and discussed at length. Conversations and support are important in all admissions whether the resident is alert or comatose. No one can tell you exactly what the comatose person understands, so you should always assume they understand what you are saying and treat their admission just as you would treat the admission of an alert resident. The nursing home social worker and charge nurse should be very helpful to the families, as well as to the resident, during any admission. Their emotional support helps allay everyone's fear and anxiety. All admissions should be well organized and planned and the prospective resident and family should be attended to by a caring thoughtful staff. Unfortunately, this is not always the case, and at least one family has told me of the inattentive, insensitive treatment they received as they were greeted at the front door of a facility. A resident once told me that she felt very uncomfortable for several days because nobody bothered to introduce her to other people. "I felt as though I was invisible until it came time to get my pills or my meal. You'd think the nursing home staff would know and remember things like this. I guess they think of us as patients and not people."

All through your preparations for the move, seek help from professionals or from others who have gone through the same experience. In my case, when my father was faced with the need for a nursing home, our family physician spoke with him, easing the burden on my family. You might speak with the nursing home's social worker or nursing staff, or ask the admissions director to refer you to people you can call on for help and suggestions. Many individuals who have placed a relative in a long-term care facility will be glad to offer advice in your time of need.

Preparations

On admissions day, you and your relative will have important paperwork to complete. You can save valuable time by doing preliminary work before admissions day: gathering information, discussing decisions your relative will have to make, and preparing lists for the administrator and the nursing staff. The more you do ahead, the more time you will be able to spend calmly helping your relative on her first day in the nursing home.

The nursing staff will need detailed information about your relative's physical condition, so I recommend that you make a list of important facts to take with you on admissions day. If the nurses know as much as possible about your relative, they can begin giving a high-quality care as soon as she is admitted.

INFORMATION TO TAKE ON ADMISSIONS DAY

- Your relative's height and weight (since medications are ordered according to weight)
- Her hearing or visual disturbances
- Any pain she experiences
- Medicines or other substances she uses, such as liniments, cough preparations, or vitamins
- Information about any aids she uses, such as a walker, crutches, cane, or wheelchair
- Her ability to get in and out of bed and to the bathroom
- Any recent trauma she has had
- Any medical condition that requires immediate attention, such as diabetes or seizures
- Any allergies or adverse reactions to medications
- Information about her pacemaker, artificial limbs or eyes, including the date of their insertion and the care they require
- Her need for oxygen, catheter care, or tube feedings
- Skin or foot conditions that require special care
- Her use of dentures, eyeglasses, or hearing aids

You should also write down the kinds of personal care you think your relative will need.

PERSONAL CARE NOTES

- Does she need help with dressing?
- Does she wash and bathe herself?
- Does she prefer a shower to a bath?
- Is she able to chew and swallow regular foods?
- Should foods be ground up to facilitate swallowing without choking?
- If she has definite food preferences, request them.
- Is she allergic to any food? This information will be sent to the dietary department.

The staff will want detailed information about your relative's behavior.

BEHAVIORAL NOTES

- Is she oriented to person, place, and time?
- Is her memory good for recent and past events?
- Is she agreeable and compliant in her daily care or does she become hostile, argumentative, and disruptive, denying her needs for such necessities as bathing and dressing?
- Does she become restless, or suffer from insomnia, lethargy, or listlessness?

Any information regarding her behavior is helpful, even though this behavior may change for better or worse over a short period of time.

MISCELLANEOUS NOTES

- Emergency numbers of neighbors or friends to be called in case a family member cannot be reached
- Religious preference, clergy, and church or synagogue affiliations
- Hospital records, if she is coming from the hospital
- Social security, private insurance, and Medicare and/or Medicaid identification cards: The admissions director should make copies of her identification cards and return the originals to you

---

There is a last—and difficult—kind of preparation to do before taking your relative to the nursing home: you should ask her about her wishes should she suffer a terminal illness while in the nursing home. It is depressing for a resident or family, especially at the time of admission, to be thinking of death; however, many admissions directors will ask for information about organ donations, living wills, and funeral home preference. If you talk about these choices ahead of time in a gentle and understanding way, you can avoid some of the trauma that a later, hasty discussion might cause.

Briefly, here are some of the issues to decide on. Does your relative wish to become an organ donor at the time of her death? If she does, she should give that information in writing to the admissions and nursing departments. Will she want to write a living will? A living will is a declaration that gives the resident a choice of whether to end treatments that prolong life or to continue everything medically possible. The will is drawn up by a resident of sound mind. If it is your relative's request to have a living will, her decision should be respected by all family members, even those who may disagree. Check with a lawyer and your state's regulations regarding the drawing up and enforcement of such a will.

Other legal matters you and your relative should consider are the powers and the durable powers of attorney. Giving someone the power of attorney will allow your relative to have legal and financial matters handled by someone other than herself. The durable power of attorney remains valid even, if and when, she becomes incompetent and may have stricter guidelines to be followed. Your relative must be of sound mind when signing the papers and must name the person she is designating. For example, if your relative names you, you will legally make all decisions regarding her finances and care.

Paperwork

All your advance preparation will shorten the time you and your relative spend on paperwork at the nursing home, but she will still have to sign major documents on admissions day. Unless she is declared incompetent, only she, rather than a third party (including a family member), can sign all the necessary papers. Who determines an individual's competency and what about the resident who is considered incompetent? There are state laws that are used to judge a person's competence. The Health Care and Financing Administration requires that a nursing home have written policies ensuring that a residents' rights pass to a guardian, next of kin, or sponsoring agency if the resident is found incompetent under state law or is determined by her physician to be incapable of understanding her rights. If your relative has been documented to be incompetent, give copies of the documents to the admissions counselor. As long as your relative has not been found incompetent, she will be expected to sign the admissions agreements and other papers herself.

All the necessary paperwork is done in English. What about the foreign-speaking prospective resident? To help her during admissions, her family should provide contact people. Members of the resident's church or synagogue may be called upon to interpret. Usually a foreign-speaking prospective resident has been under the care of a doctor who speaks her language, and the doctor may be contacted for help. Some area colleges have students who are anxious to use their newfound foreign language skills and may be of assistance with the elderly. Also helpful are members of the American Association of Retired Persons (see Appendix D for other resources).

Any forms you or your relative are asked to sign during admission should be ones with which you are familiar. Nursing homes are careful about this but it is always to your advantage to check before signing anything.

What to Bring, What to Leave at Home

During the years I've spent in nursing homes, I've come to know which items new residents should bring and which ones they shouldn't. Some possessions are better left at home simply because they won't be used, but others, such as cigarette lighters, razor blades, sharp scissors, or flammable pillows, should be left because they present a danger. One thing is especially important: label everything. You can use sew-in labels, laundry markers, indelible pens, or tape, but be sure each item (and each removable part such as the footrests on a wheelchair) has your relative's name on it.

On admission day, everything your relative brings will be listed on a personal item record which she and her charge nurse will sign. Each time an item is brought in or removed, the personal list is updated and signed by both the family (or the resident) and the nurse.

Mrs. G., who at times was confused, could not locate a blue nightgown that she said her daughter had brought in on the previous day. The nurse quickly referred to the personal items list to verify that the family member did indeed bring in a nightgown that day, and without having to contact the family for information, she found the article of clothing in Mrs. G.'s roommate's closet.

The nurses quickly learn of favorite hiding places on the unit and will look there before calling the families.

Bring your relative's clothing and personal items with you

on admissions day. Clothes most easily managed by the elderly have Velcro fasteners, as opposed to snaps or hooks and eyes. We sometimes forget how difficult it is to handle small zipper pulls! Imagine a resident's distress if she continually has difficulty with zippers. Encourage your relative to help you decide how to alter her clothing for easier dressing. Nightgowns with front ties are easier to handle than ones that require lifting up both arms and pulling over the head. If your relative is bed bound, it will be easier for the nursing staff if her gowns have ties in the back. Hospital gowns are made this way and are available in many different patterns and colors (check with medical supply companies and local department stores). Don't forget cotton underpants and pantyhose with cotton crotches. Discourage the use of garters as they constrict blood flow. In many cases, men find that their trousers are held up more easily by suspenders than by belts. Even women sometimes prefer using suspenders. Loose fitting pants are more comfortable for both men and women and suspenders can be invaluable. Long-handled shoe horns are another useful tool for both male and female residents.

Favorite personal items that residents like to bring include comforters, soft and warm blankets, lap robes, shawls, and lambswool lined slippers. Lambswool mattress covers which can be bought at local department stores or through the nursing home's medical supply firm provide for extra padding and comfort. Some residents who enjoy reading in bed like soft bed-rest pillows. Since most sleeping pillows at nursing homes are not very comfortable, bring in your own soft pillow.

Footrests and ottomans may help your relative relax and reduce the swelling of her feet. If your footrest or ottoman is stuffed, it should be checked by the maintenance department for nonflammable content. If your relative has a television she wants to bring, this will also be checked for safety. Another item enjoyed by all is the small stereo radio with earphones for private listening.

Bring a clock with large numerals, and a radio. A nonslip mat for these items is a nice addition to the nightstand. Lamps are provided by the nursing home and nightlights are also a part of the resident's room. Nonslip shower and bath mats are provided as standard items. If you plan to regularly do your relative's laundry, bring a covered laundry container on admission day.

While some facilities allow residents to hang framed pictures, each home has its own policy regarding this, so it is necessary to check with the director of admissions before hanging anything. Do bring photo albums and favorite small pictures.

Something new in nursing homes since the inception of VCRs is the videotape of the resident with her relatives. These tapes, brought in by the resident or her family, are proving to be invaluable in alleviating agitation and aggressive behavior. In one nursing home, when Mrs. Wills began crying for her husband, the staff put her cassette tape into the VCR and showed her movies that had been taken in the past of her, her husband, and other family members. If they continue to be successful, nursing home personnel may find less need to give tranquilizers during periods of a resident's distress. If you have family videos, consider taking them along to the nursing home.

Be sure to bring personal items your relative needs, such as eyeglasses (labeled with the resident's name on adhesive tape on the bow), a specially lighted magnifying glass, and a hearing aid. Hearing-aid batteries are small and easy to misplace; they can be kept at the nurse's station. Other immediate needs of some new residents are canes, walkers, or wheelchairs. Although facilities will offer short-term use of walking aids, there is often a shortage of such items, so it is wise to bring your relative's own.

There are some items the nursing staff may ask you not to bring. Any form of medicine, either brought from a hospital or from home, including even innocuous over-the-counter ointments, nose drops, cough medicines, vitamins, rubbing compounds, and arthritis medications, can become quite dangerous if picked up and swallowed by another resident. The rule that all medications and ointments should be kept at the nurse's station provides a safety factor for residents. Family members will often say, "But Mother is so alert and capable of taking her own medications." This may well be the case, but the nursing home cannot assume that all the other residents are so alert. There are residents who may take their own medications, according to a new federal regulation, but a doctor's order is required for any resident to keep any medicines in their room.

Heating pads not specifically ordered by a physician and checked by the engineer for safety should not be brought without consulting the nurse. Overstuffed chairs should be checked by the engineer for flammability before they are allowed in. Do not bring expensive jewelry; instead, buy inexpensive costume jewelry. A doctor's order is necessary before bringing any alcoholic beverages. If your relative is accustomed to a glass of wine before dinner, you may want to request the order for this from the nurse during admission. Some nursing homes won't allow scissors, matches, and lighters to be kept in the residents' rooms, but they may be borrowed from the nurse as needed.

The First Day

I have always found that midmorning is the best time to bring your relative for admission. Its's a good idea to call ahead and tell the nurse that you are on your way. If she knows when to expect you, she can allot ample time for orientation to the facility.

Usually the admissions director or social worker will meet you and your relative and provide you with needed documents, such as the patient's Bill of Rights, the nursing home's policies, and its financial requirements. At this time, she may ask you for details about your relative's health, personality, and needs. You can give her the lists and the information you wrote earlier.

If your relative has a tendency to wander, tell the admissions director and social worker before they take her up to her unit. In some nursing homes, a special arm bracelet, which will set off an alarm if she should wander out of doors, will be provided.

If your relative frequently wakes up for a snack during the night, tell the staff so they can make the necessary provisions. Minor accommodations to a resident's needs help to make the adjustment period easier.

Mr. W., a ninety-year-old-man, would get up in the middle of the night to look for a snack. We had been informed by his family of his nightly routine when he was in strange places. So the first night he appeared at the nurses' station, the staff was prepared. Still half asleep, he went to the refrigerator, got a glass of milk and a few cookies, and walked over to the sitting room. He switched on the television and sat there until he could no longer keep his head up. Occasionally he would glance in our direction as though to assure himself that he was not alone. When he eventually drifted off to sleep, we gently put him into a comfortable position and rested his head on a pillow, and there he remained, content that someone was watching over him. Night after night this routine continued, as though an internal alarm always awakened him at the same hour. One night the hour passed and no Mr. W. We raced quickly back to his room, afraid of what we would find, and there, snoring away, was Mr. W. We set a glass of milk along with a few cookies on his nightstand and quietly tiptoed out. That was the last time we saw Mr. W. in the middle of the night. He slept through each night thereafter without waking (or at least without coming out to the nursing station). However, the cookies and milk were always gone in the morning! He would not admit to eating the cookies; rather, he said, "The cookie monster must've eaten them." Mr. W. was secure in knowing that we were always there.

After your meeting with the admissions counselor or social worker, you and your relative will be taken to the nursing unit and introduced to the charge nurse. She will try to make your relative feel very much at home and will ask how she likes to be addressed; some residents prefer first names while others like full names. The nurse will give your relative an armband imprinted with her name, room number, and physician, and will place the physician's name and phone number in her room. The nurse will also provide any necessary personal care items that you may have forgotten.

Next, the charge nurse may ask detailed questions concerning your relative's needs, especially her bowel routine. Elimination needs are of major concern to residents since the elderly have definite routines that should be followed if at all possible. The nurse may ask if your relative uses laxatives or enemas routinely. She will ask if your relative has a colostomy (an artificial rectal opening on the abdomen) and will want to know which products are being used in its care. She will assist you in checking personal items for indelible labels. She will also label your relative's door, bed, and closet. Then she will assign her to a specific nursing assistant who will orient her to the unit and introduce her to others. During this introduction time, the nurse will take the hospital or personal records that you have brought, discuss various aspects of your relative's needs and care, and tell you about visiting hours and telephone calls during the adjustment period to the nursing home.

If your relative smokes, tell the nurse now. Smoking areas in a nursing home are restricted, and matches are not provided to a resident at any time. She can get a light for her cigarette from the nurse. Of course, smoking is prohibited in a patient's room. A resident who refuses to comply with the nursing home's policies on smoking can be asked to leave the facility permanently.

If you have any questions, ask them now, and if your family member is alert and oriented to her surroundings, encourage her to ask and answer questions on her own.

When Mrs. D. was asked questions about her personal care, her family was very helpful in answering for her. Mrs. D. sat very quietly for several minutes and then looked up at the nurse. She said, "My daughter doesn't know that I can still think for myself and answer questions even though I'm going into a nursing home." She chuckled, as everyone smiled at her.

Mrs. D. was amused at the situation but it can be extremely upsetting to a new resident not to be allowed to answer for herself.

At the time of admission, you may remain with your relative as long as you desire. However, you should be aware that some residents become very upset when their families leave. Emotional upsets are not uncommon and in most cases subside. Nursing home personnel should be well trained in the care of the resident during this period, and they will advise you on the best way to minimize stress on all.

Adjustments

You can never tell in advance just how your loved one is going to react to entering a nursing home. For some new residents, adjustment seems to be a simple matter of finding out where things are and when things happen. For others, the change is, at best, difficult. Mrs. R. was upset when she found out the routine of the nursing home allowed for a bath twice a week. The schedule was rearranged so that she would take her daily bath. Other residents don't want to eat in a large main dining room but want all meals in their own room. The nursing home's routine may be different than what a resident is used to and, when possible, may have to be changed to fit an individual's needs. When the staff of a nursing home is concerned with the quality of a resident's life, they are sure to provide all the emotional support necessary to allay the resident's and her family's anxieties.

It's not unusual for a new resident to feel any number of stress-related symptoms, from a slight nervousness to outright hostility. In some exaggerated cases, new residents have suffered from delusions and hallucinations. These cases, though, are the exception.

However, in many cases, the symptoms of stress make the new resident "feel plain awful." Sometimes stress appears as a loss of appetite, an increase in blood pressure, an upset stomach, or other usually minor complaints.

The geriatric nurse, adept at helping to resolve residents' conflicts, spends time with a new resident, trying to explain bodily changes and relocation stress. She explains that this is common to all new residents, and she may suggest that your relative talk with others who have successfully adjusted to their new home. She will carefully weigh how much to tell the new resident during admission and how much can be talked about at a later time. When families recall the day of admission to the nursing home, most say that it was an emotional blur and they remember only half of what was told them on that day. The social worker also comes and talks to your relative about the transition that has taken place and makes suggestions to minimize stress. Additionally, the activities director is available to involve her in a meaningful activity, if that is her choice. The resident's clergy may visit at this time and can be helpful in providing emotional comfort and support.

If your relative is extremely agitated and has rejected all forms of external diversion, the nurse may call the physician for a temporary order for a tranquilizer, which provides mild sedation. In cases such as these, when a resident is so emotionally upset, a few days on a tranquilizer are usually all that is needed. Within these few days the resident usually adjusts to the nursing home routine and begins to benefit from the support services that are offered.

The adjustment period can be very trying for the resident's family as well. You may feel an overwhelming sense of guilt over placing your relative in a nursing home.

You may feel that you must call the nursing home frequently to inquire about all aspects of your loved one's condition. However, difficulties and stress can be caused by frequent family calls to the resident. You may mean well, but your relative's best interests will be served by following the direction of those who are trained in geriatrics. Phone calls to your relative should be kept to a minimum during the first few days and should be made only to ask what you might bring and to remind her of your love.

During this period of emotional unrest, the nurse may suggest that you and your family make an appointment with the social worker to discuss any guilt feelings you may have. Feelings of guilt must be recognized and dealt with; there is a high price for denying guilt. Frustration, insomnia, and marital discord can all follow extreme stress. Sometimes a family may even reject the nursing home resident in order to cope with their own distress. Yet, denying the emotional needs of the resident is most harmful and can even turn into overt neglect. The social worker, with her expertise and training, can help you understand that your feelings are quite normal and will eventually subside. She may even suggest that you call on other residents' family members or talk to other families when they come to visit.

Families of residents with Alzheimer's disease are especially upset at this time. They worry about who will call them if their relative is upset, wanders away, or is in pain. They want to know how anyone else could possibly know that when "Mother paces the floor, it usually means she has to go to the bathroom." They want to know how they can communicate with the doctor or how the doctor will communicate with their mother. Families are also afraid that their questions sound unintelligent. Constant reassurance should be given to the family at all times, but especially during this emotional period. The staff of a nursing home concerned with the residents' quality of life will remind the family that everyone will be working together for the well-being of the resident.

The resident, if she is able to communicate her fears, may say she is afraid that her family will desert her. She may have heard, or seen, others who were neglected, and she may now feel that she too will be left without a family to care for, visit, and look out for her welfare. She should be reassured that the family will visit as often as possible. In most cases, no one intentionally neglects a relative who has been admitted to a nursing facility. There are a variety of reasons why a family may not visit frequently. Some family members never learn to cope with the guilt they feel; others simply cannot accept old age as part of the life cycle. They think of their relative as she once was and cannot accept this stage of her life. There are also those who prefer not to be reminded that the nursing home may be part of their own future living situation. Some families are separated by great distances and cannot visit as often as they would like. Lastly, and sadly, there are those family relationships that have been emotionally strained and never happy. In these cases, visits from the family may be few and far between.

Many adjustments take place after admission to a nursing home. Not all individuals react in negative ways; sometimes the resident who was a "reigning terror" at home, never satisfied, always demanding, and even hostile to friends when they occasionally visited, on admission becomes a cooperative, pleasant, unassuming, and considerate individual. One may wonder, "What happened to cause this change in behavior?" Did you ever stop to think of the pressure that an eighty-year-old is under trying to conform to an environment with which she no longer has anything in common—living a life that, for her, no longer exists?

She may see her younger and healthier friends out walking, shopping, and socializing, and it becomes a constant reminder to her that she cannot keep up, that she is playing a part that is much too difficult and stressful to her. Her mind is filled with memories of her past, and she is aware that those days are gone forever. Living in this way causes undue stress and can lead to all types of unusual behavior. When she is relieved of this stress by being admitted to a nursing home where she is around others her age and in similar situations, she knows that she can finally relax and be herself. She no longer must prove to herself and others that she can continue on as she once did. She has found her new home.

The move to a nursing home can be a very emotional time for the new resident as well as her family. The most important thing to remember is: you are not alone and any feelings of guilt and anxiety should be acknowledged and dealt with. The geriatric facility is staffed by professionals who are trained to care for your relative whether she is alert and oriented or suffering from cognitive impairment. If you have further questions and concerns, I urge you to discuss them before you leave the home. And lastly, remember: you have looked at and compared other nursing homes and chosen the one that you feel offers the best possible care for your relative. Now it is time for the professional staff to do their job to the best of their ability.

6

Living in a Nursing Home

During my years as a geriatric nurse, I have talked to many families about their concerns and uncertainties. Some of the questions I've been asked are specific to individual cases. Most everyone has the same concerns and questions about their relatives' health, comfort, recovery, and future. Families want to know about the everyday health problems their relatives will face and about how the nursing home will handle emergencies. Residents ask about the problem of chronic, severe pain. Many families ask how to improve their own relationships with their relatives and what to bring when they visit. Finally, they want to know what to expect if their relative wants to go to another nursing home. In this chapter, I will share the questions I am most commonly asked and give you the best answers I can based on my medical and personal experience. Not all the information I give you will work in all cases. Use it as a starting point or as a general guide.

Everyday Medical Problems

Q: My relative just entered the nursing home and is losing weight. Why?

A: Although it may seem worrisome, weight loss or fluctuation is not unusual immediately after admission. Over the years, your relative has gotten used to the cooking he had at home and now, in his new environment, he has to get used to the nursing home's food. Most facilities have appetizing meals served attractively, but nothing is ever like home. It may take him a while to adjust, but his weight will probably stabilize within several weeks, if it is not part of a chronic, debilitating disease. The doctor will be kept informed of your relative's weight.

Q: I'm afraid that my mother will pick up infections in the nursing home. Should I worry?

A: Good nursing homes try everything possible to keep infections from spreading. However, infections can occur easily in older people because their immune systems are sometimes drastically weakened. Certain diseases can also make the elderly more prone to infections. The most perplexing problem of infection in the elderly is diagnosis. Their symptoms are not as clearly defined as young people's and they may have a confusing mixture of complaints. Many times an elderly individual is not able to talk about her discomfort. Instead, nurses have to look for signs of infection. Changes in facial features and expressions, confusion, a difference in behavior, increased listlessness, insomnia, agitation and argumentative behavior, and increased pacing of the floor are some of the symptoms of infection in the elderly.

Here are some of the common infections found in nursing homes:

Flu: There are seasonal flu and virus epidemics that can seriously affect nursing homes. Some facilities restrict visitors other than the residents' immediate families, during flu season.

Pneumonia: This lung condition can be the result of bacterial infections, occur as a result of a cold, or be due to prolonged immobilization. In some cases, pneumonia can also be caused by choking on food or fluid (this is called "aspiration pneumonia").

Prostatitis: This mild inflammation of the prostate gland is a common infection of elderly men. At times it can lead to high fever and kidney infection.

Vaginitis: This is a common problem in elderly women and may cause vaginal bleeding and irritation. It is sometimes associated with yeast infections that come after recent use of antibiotics. Vaginitis can also be caused by bacteria that gain entrance from a local skin irritation. Some residents say nylon panties cause chafing and irritation, especially in hot weather. Bladder infections can be confused with vaginitis because the symptoms may be similar.

Shingles (herpes zoster): This is caused by the same virus that causes chickenpox in children, and its symptoms include pain, itching, a red rash with raised areas resembling bubbles filled with fluid, and a severe form of neuralgia (pain along a nerve path).

Urinary Tract Infections: These can occur in the elderly for various reasons and can cause an increased urge to void and burning on urination.

While you are right to be concerned about infection, there is no need for excessive worrying if your relative's nursing home follows procedures to reduce the spread of infection.

Q: Should I ask the doctor to prescribe a flu shot for my relative?

A: Before flu season, the charge nurse should call the residents' physicians to get orders for flu shots. She will get permission, from either your relative or you before giving the shot.

Q: The nurse says my father has edema. What is that?

A: Edema is an accumulation of fluid in the tissues and is seen frequently in the feet and ankles. Your father may notice a little swelling after a day of walking or sitting in a chair with his feet hanging down. His ankles and feet may swell, his shoes may fit too tightly, and his skin may appear shiny. The edema should subside when he raises and rests his feet for a while. For a person confined to a chair all day, an ottoman is invaluable. If edema persists beyond two or three days and there is a dramatic increase in your relative's weight, or if your relative has a heart problem, the physician may order a diuretic (a pill that rids the tissues of excess fluid) for a few days. There are other causes of edema but not all swelling is a sign of serious illness.

Q: What causes my mother's frequent urinary tract infections?

A: Urinary tract infections are common, especially among female residents. They can be caused by improper cleansing after bowel movements, or irritation from a catheter. If your relative has a catheter, check with the staff to be sure she is cleansed several times a day with antibacterial agents, that her drainage bag is kept clean, and that the drainage tubing is not kinked. If she has pain while urinating or has blood in her urine, her doctor will most likely order a urinalysis, a urine culture, and, when needed, an antibiotic.

Q: What can be done about my relative's constipation?

A: Constipation might be due to inactivity and lack of exercise. Elimination troubles are also associated with lack of fluid or bulk foods in the diet. The nursing home staff will try to help your relative by giving him extra fluids and an exercise program. However, since many residents are not used to a formal exercise class, your relative may need some persuasion before he attends. The dietitian may try some bran in his cereal and warm prune juice in the morning.

Q: What causes pressure sores and how are they treated?

A: Pressure sores are one of the most dreaded problems in nursing homes. They are a particular problem for those who are bed-bound, are confined to a wheelchair or geriatric chair, are incontinent, or have nutritional, metabolic, or circulatory problems. Anything that interferes with blood circulation to an area of the body or causes excess friction can cause pressure sores. Wrinkled sheets are another cause of reddened pressure areas.

Your relative's nurse should check all the residents carefully at bathing time and ask for daily reports from her nursing assistants about residents' skin conditions. She should especially be on the lookout for pressure sores on those who have elevated temperatures and other signs of illness.

All precautions should be taken to avoid pressure and skin breakdown. Lambswool "bunny boots" protect the bony prominences of the feet and ankles, and elbow pads protect against friction from bed sheets. Any bony prominence should be given extra protection. A resident confined to bed and unable to turn herself should be turned and positioned comfortably every two hours by the nurse. Shifts in body weight and position, even small ones, alleviate constant pressure and redness.

A good foam egg-crate mattress, wheelchair or bed pad, air or water mattress are invaluable in the care of a bed-confined resident. When preventive care does not solve the problem of pressure and a resident's skin breaks down, there are several methods of treatment, ranging from the simple to the complex and all ordered by the physician. The doctor may also order extra protein, calories, and vitamins in the diet to aid the rebuilding of body tissue.

Disease and Disability

Q: If there is an emergency, what hospital will my relative be taken to?

A: If your relative is acutely ill or severely injured, the rescue squad will take him to the closest hospital. The most important thing at such a time is to get him to the hospital quickly, provide emergency care, and then, only after treatment, discuss a transfer to another hospital by private ambulance.

For nonemergency admissions, you and your relative can choose a hospital. The primary physician should be informed of your choice before your relative's admission to the nursing home, for the doctor may not be on the staff of the hospital you select or may prefer not to use that hospital. However, the nursing home and the doctor should do what they can to accommodate your request.

After your relative is treated, and depending on his condition, he may return to the nursing home.

Q: If my relative needs emergency surgery and I am out of town, will I be notified before the surgery?

A: Before going out of town, always leave an emergency number where you can be reached. Also, you should give the nursing home a list of relatives who can be called in your absence. This is especially important if you are a frequent traveler. Keep in mind that a resident who is coherent and of sound mind is responsible for the acceptance or refusal of any or all treatments.

Q: Can I see my relative's records?

A: Your relative may obtain a record of anything that has been done for her during her hospitalization or nursing home stay. Complete copies of the file can be obtained through the facility's medical records department or she can read the record and ask for a copy of just the necessary information.

Rules regarding access to medical records vary in different facilities, but all residents have a right to know about their diagnosis, treatment, plan of care, and prognosis.

Q: My father has Alzheimer's disease. Are there special programs for him?

A: The Office of Technology Assessment, in Washington,

D.C., can put you in touch with 150 programs for Alzheimer's patients. Inquire at any facility you are considering to see if it has a special unit for a resident with Alzheimer's disease. Also contact the Alzheimer's Disease and Related Disorders Association (ADRDA) for invaluable help, information, referrals, and support.

Q: Does Medicaid provide special benefits to the nursing home for the care of my relative with Alzheimer's disease?

A: Until recently, some facilities were known to refuse admission to a patient with Alzheimer's disease because they lacked adequately trained staff and state-funded Medicaid to cover the extra care involved. The U.S. Senate Special Committee on Aging reported this discriminatory act and found that patients with Alzheimer's disease were often in hospitals waiting for beds even when there were nursing home beds available. A patient with Alzheimer's disease can be extremely difficult to care for; her emotional and physical needs are many. While state Medicaid funding may allow for extra services to meet your relative's physical needs, it unfortunately does not pay for the trained staffing required to meet her emotional needs.

Q: Why does my relative need protective devices?

A: These devices are used to protect your relative from danger to himself or others. A protective device may be necessary if a resident is not able to walk unassisted and his attempts to do so have led to frequent falls and injuries. One protective device is a vest with straps to comfortably secure a resident to either a chair or a bed. A geriatric chair, one equipped with a tray that can be locked in a lap position, is of use in keeping some residents from wandering unassisted. Wrist and ankle devices can be used on extremely agitated residents or those in need of intravenous feedings who, if left unrestrained, would pull out the intravenous needle and thereby cause injury. If your relative uses any protective device, be sure that it is loosened regularly and that your relative is repositioned every two hours.

There is another type of restraint used in nursing homes: chemical restraint, using medications such as tranquilizers to quiet excessive agitation in residents. While chemical restraint has a place, a nursing home should not use drugs inappropriately or when other methods of calming residents would work as well.

Since new federal regulations discourage the use of restraints, many nursing homes are beginning to change their attitudes about the necessity of these devices. Previously, to prevent falls in one who was unsteady when walking, a protective device may have been used as soon as the resident got out of bed in the morning. Now it is more common to see the residents being assisted in walking, helped into a comfortable easy chair, and included in many more activities than it is to see residents tied to a chair and left there to sit without any activity level for hours.

Some nursing homes are even referring to their new policy of "restraint-free care." You may wonder if this is possible. Studies have shown that some residents who are unsteady when walking may fall more when left unrestrained; however, it could happen that these same residents would also fall out of bed or a chair if they were struggling to untie a protective device. The answer must be to do whatever is best for the resident and enhances his quality of life. It is believed that it is more important in a resident's daily life to be encouraged to walk and mingle with other residents than to be overly concerned about falls that may or may not occur.

Some of the residents who had been restrained for long periods of time were those who were also heavily medicated with tranquilizers. With new federal regulations ensuring a decreased use of tranquilizers and restraints, a higher quality of life can be expected in the nation's nursing homes.

Q: Will I be notified if my relative hits or injures someone?

A: Yes, families are notified just as though the resident herself had been the one injured. If your relative injures another, she may be asked to leave the facility without notice. This is also the case if she sets a fire or does anything that would endanger the safety of others.

Q: My relative has Parkinson's disease and is being admitted to a nursing home. Is there anything special that I should be aware of?

A: Nursing homes are very familiar with the care of residents with Parkinson's disease. There are two types of

Parkinson's: the primary and the drug-induced varieties. In some cases, drug-induced Parkinson's can often be reversed by stopping the medications, such as strong tranquilizers, that bring on the symptoms.

Parkinson's can be a debilitating disease. As it progresses, your relative will begin to develop tremors of his head and extremities, lose his facial expressions, and develop a fixed stare. He will still experience emotions even though his face will show no sign of feeling. As time goes by, he may become depressed and experience severe motor disturbances. Physically, he will develop a stooped-over posture associated with difficulty in walking.

The patient with Parkinson's disease suffers a decrease in the brain's dopamine (a chemical that transmits nerve impulses). One treatment is to give medications that restore the level of dopamine in the brain.

The National Institute of Neurological and Communicative Disorders and Stroke, at National Institutes of Health, Bethesda, Maryland, is the major source of support for research on the causes and treatments of this disease. You can contact them for information on treatment and local organizations.

Q: The nurses talk about strokes and TIAs. What are they referring to?

A: TIA stands for transient-ischemic attack and is a temporary lack of oxygen to a part of the brain, resulting in minor symptoms such as dizziness, a brief loss of memory, an unsteady gait, and ringing in the ears. The significance of a TIA is its relationship to larger, impending strokes. Larger strokes do not always occur and many TIAs pass uneventfully, only to recur.

Q: My relative has had a stroke. What can the nursing home do for her?

A: A stroke (or CVA—cerebrovascular accident) results from blood clots, hemorrhage, or blockage of blood vessels in the brain, which can cause paralysis, speech and sight disturbances, and damage to the senses. If your relative has suffered from a massive stroke, she may require the care given to a bed-confined resident, including having her meals fed her by a nursing assistant or given through a tube. She may also be incontinent and need a catheter or absorbent pads and an egg-crate mattress and chair pad to keep her skin from breaking down.

Aside from physical care, your relative will need therapy to help her regain her abilities. The nursing home's physical therapist will help get your relative moving to prevent deformities, and try to retrain her to walk.

If your relative's speech was affected by the stroke, she may have aphasia, which is an inability to express her needs and wants. When she tries to say a certain word, an entirely different word may come out, much to her distress. This can be very frightening and frustrating.

Speech therapy may restore speech, but in some cases this is not possible, depending on the type and severity of the stroke. The entire recovery process can be very lengthy and may seriously depress your relative. Constant encouragement and support from the nursing staff will help her recovery.

For more information, contact your local office of the Easter Seal Foundation, which provides lists of stroke clubs, and the American Heart Association which offers a booklet of self-help devices your relative can use.

Q: My father has a pacemaker. Will this be taken care of at the nursing home?

A: While pacers require no special nursing care, you should let the nurse know when the pacemaker was implanted and how your father checks its operation. Pacer checks might be done by telephone at the nursing home.

Q: My mother, who is terminally ill, is a recovering alcoholic. Can her AA group hold meetings at the nursing home and visit with her?

A: Most facilities will allow someone from AA to visit and counsel your relative. As for group meetings, discuss this with your nursing home administrator.

Q: My relative is blind. Are nursing home activities geared to the sight-impaired also?

A: There are many activities that the blind can participate in, such as group sing-a-longs, walks with the assistance of a volunteer, picnics and celebrations, and group discussions. Local libraries have talking books that can be checked out for the blind resident. In addition, you can contact the American Foundation for the Blind, 15 West 16th Street,

New York, New York 10011, and request information and the location of local support groups. They will send you numerous brochures on what is available for the blind. Activities directors know about resource materials and are particularly good at discovering the hidden talents and interests of the handicapped.

Pain Control

Q: My relative has severe arthritis. How can his pain be controlled?

A: A variety of techniques, used in combination, can help your relative with his arthritis pain. A common way of treating arthritis pain is with medication. For certain types of arthritis, the drug of choice for many years has been aspirin in very large doses. However, aspirin can be very irritating to the stomach and must be given with food. Over a period of time, your relative may have increasing arthritis pain that is unrelieved by huge doses of aspirin. When this occurs, his doctor will try different antiarthritic medications.

Pain can also be controlled through "nursing measures" such as proper body alignment, perhaps with the use of pillows; immobilization with splints and neck braces (for certain types of activities); and hot or cold packs. Physical therapy is extremely important to residents who have severe arthritis. In the physical therapy program, your relative will do exercises to prevent "frozen" joints and contractures. Massage and whirlpool can also help alleviate pain.

Another technique that may help your relative is transcutaneous electrical nerve stimulation (TENS). Because TENS is narcotic-free and noninvasive, it is popular with physicians.

If all else fails and your relative is in excruciating pain and unresponsive to medication, he may need surgery to relieve the contractures associated with severe cases of arthritis.

The National Institute of Arthritis, Diabetes, Digestive and Kidney Disease can give you the latest information on the treatment of arthritis pain. You can write them at the National Institutes of Health, Bethesda, MD 20205.

Q: My relative has cancer. What can we do about her pain?

A: Cancer, in its terminal stage, can cause different types and degrees of pain, depending on the location of the tumor and the degree to which it has spread. If a tumor has displaced organs from their normal position, pressure from these organs exerted on nerves will cause pain. Some residents will complain of a dull, constant, boring type of pain. Others complain of shortness of breath and pain associated with deep breaths. Some terminal cancer patients experience no pain, or at least say they are pain-free. The question is not what type of pain your relative has, but how she can be kept as comfortable as possible.

Pain relief for someone who has cancer and a life expectancy of several years can present a challenge even to the most knowledgeable physicians. When my father was diagnosed with cancer, the doctor recommended that his pain medication be given only when he was extremely uncomfortable. In this way, he would be kept free of addiction for as long as possible. The latest thoughts are that the quality of a person's remaining life is more important than whether she uses addictive, pain-relieving medications. Your doctor should prescribe pain-relieving medications that will enable your relative to participate in activities that give her enjoyment or add meaning to her life. Some of the medications that do this, other than pain killers, are tranquilizers and mood elevators.

In years past, nurses would wait until a resident requested medication before giving it. However, this method did not keep the resident pain-free. The practice today is for the nurse to obtain an order that reads, "Give medication every four hours," dropping the "as needed" caveat.

The nurses should continually monitor your relative for signs of pain. She may grimace and decrease her activity level or lose her appetite, become restless, pace, and suffer from insomnia. If the nurse suspects that your relative is experiencing a great degree of pain, she will call the doctor to discuss stronger medication.

One drug introduced in the United States that has been used in England for many years is a pain-relieving medical "cocktail" consisting of a narcotic, a stimulant, alcohol, and flavoring. This combination not only provides pain relief but may allow your relative to remain alert and participate in activities.

There is a newer method of pain relief called patient-controlled analgesia, or PCA. PCA is self-administered through a needle in the patient's body which is hooked up to a pump. Its advantages are: better relief using a lower dosage, less drowsiness, and no waiting for a doctor or nurse to give the medication. Less worry over adequate pain control seems to be the biggest advantage of its use, as the patient can regulate its use according to the severity of pain. The pump automatically adjusts the amount of medicine to prevent overdosage. This method of pain control may be seen in nursing homes more often in the future.

Q: How do the nurses keep semicomatose and nonresponsive residents comfortable?

A: The nonresponsive patient is a challenge because he cannot indicate pain or other discomfort. In these cases, the nurse relies on the resident's diagnosis for clues to the discomfort he may be feeling. Other signs are grimaces, rigid muscles, excess perspiration, and constant movement.

My own father had slipped into a coma due to kidney failure in the terminal stages of his cancer. The nursing staff felt that his injections for pain were no longer necessary, since he could not feel any pain. My question was, "How do you know that?" No one could answer. He had been on injections for pain every one-to-two hours before lapsing into the coma. I was very relieved when the doctor agreed to give him pain medication at this stage whether he needed it or not.

I have always been leery of anyone who says, "Oh, he's not having any pain." If a resident says he is in pain, we must react to his feelings. Whether the pain is real or imagined, it affects his life, and quality of life is the issue in nursing homes.

Supplemental Medical Services

Q: Can I have my relative's prescriptions filled at my own pharmacy?

A: State and federal regulations govern the labeling and delivery of drugs to a nursing home. In most cases it may be necessary to use the pharmacy on contract with the nursing home. All medicines come from the nursing home's supplier in sealed containers or packages and are delivered to meet the home's scheduled needs. If emergency medications are needed, twenty-four-hour coverage is provided by the pharmacy. Some nursing homes will accept medications if the family brings them in sealed packages.

Occasionally, a resident's case is under study at the National Institutes of Health or other specialty hospital. When the resident needs particular study medications, the hospital will provide them.

If you feel strongly about using your own pharmacy— perhaps because you would feel more comfortable knowing that a familiar pharmacist is filling your relative's prescriptions—check with the director of nurses. She can tell you about the nursing home's policy and your state's regulations.

Q: Does the nursing home's pharmacist double-check the medications my relative takes?

A: The pharmacist checks physicians' orders monthly, according to federal rules and regulations. He checks that the orders are copied correctly by the charge nurse and that no errors have been made in any step of record-keeping. In addition, the pharmacist checks combinations of medicines that doctors have ordered and new orders that have been written in the past month. He also makes suggestions to the doctors and nurses about when to give medications.

Certain medications, such as antibiotics and cough medicines, may have an automatic "stop time." This means that unless a doctor has ordered otherwise, the medicine is automatically discontinued by the pharmacist after a certain amount of time. For instance, if a physician orders a cough medicine for a resident with an upper respiratory infection, the automatic stop time ensures that the resident will not receive the cough medicine beyond the usual seven to ten days without a new order.

The pharmacist also may oversee the medicine stocked in the nursing home. Stocks are kept to a minimum but may include such items as bronchodilators (to alleviate breathing distress), antibiotics, antinausea medication, suppositories for fevers (used when a resident cannot take an oral drug), heart medications, sleep medications, diuretics, and certain pain medications. The pharmacist checks expiration dates of stock medications, checks the lock on the emergency boxes of medications, and always sees that narcotics are kept under a double lock and key. He may hold training meetings for the staff to discuss new medications.

Q: **Can my relative get laboratory, X-ray, podiatry, and dental services at the nursing home?**

A: These services are provided on a consultant basis in most facilities, but some large nursing homes do have their own specialty departments. Laboratory, X-ray, podiatry, and dental services are all billed as extra charges. Podiatric care can be expensive; however, it is especially necessary for diabetics, who develop skin infections very easily, and for residents with poor circulation. Nurses do not routinely cut the toenails of residents with diabetes because of the risks.

If you want your relative to be seen by the dentist or the podiatrist, your relative needs an order from the doctor. The podiatrist usually visits on a routine basis but dental and eye exams may be done at outside offices unless a facility has its own.

Either you or the nursing home will provide the necessary transportation to outside offices. Some nursing homes own their own vans, while others call on the services of vans used by the elderly in the community. You might have neighbors and friends who will help with transportation. Keep in mind that if someone other than the family will be taking your relative out of the facility the charge nurse should be informed.

Q: **What is a drug holiday?**

A: A drug holiday is a rest from all medications except those that are absolutely necessary (such as antiseizure medications, antidiabetic drugs, and pain medicines). A physician writes the order for a drug holiday, which can occur on Saturdays and/or Sundays. Most residents look forward to these days as a time to purge their systems of accumulated drugs and as a break from routine. However, some residents do not want a rest from medication, and it is their right to continue with their medicines.

The Resident and the Family

Q: **Our family has to move out of state. Should we transfer our relative to a nursing home near our new location?**

A: This is a hard decision for you and your relative to make. There are several factors to consider. Is she content in her present nursing home? Has she developed a close relationship with others at the nursing home? How long did it take her to adjust to this new way of living? How long has she been in the facility? Would she be emotionally upset if she had to move? How often do you visit now and how often would you be able to visit from your new home? What is your relative's physical condition?

Discuss the situation with your relative's attending physician, charge nurse, or director of nurses before talking to your relative. However, keep in mind that the choice will ultimately be hers, providing she is of sound mind and in charge of her own affairs.

Q: May I take my relative on an extended vacation with the family?

A: Everyone looks on a vacation as a welcome change in routine. Residents of nursing homes are no exception. If you would like to take your relative on a trip, talk to the charge nurse, who will call the physician. If the doctor agrees to the vacation, the nurse will order the necessary medications from the pharmacy and write a schedule for you to follow. If your relative is on Medicaid, there is a limit to the number of days she may be away from the facility each year. If she is on Medicare, check with the staff before taking her out of the facility to ensure continued Medicare coverage.

Q: What should I bring when I visit my relative in the nursing home?

A: The most valuable parts of a visit are quiet conversation, hand holding, and good listening—gifts that help to convey respect and love. Think of visits you receive from your friends; what makes them so enjoyable? The visit to your relative in a nursing home should be like a visit to a friend or relative at home.

Some people feel more comfortable when they bring a gift when visiting. Baskets filled with a combination of items such as powder, perfume, after-shave lotion, magazines, and fingernail polish make nice gifts. One family brought in washable tennis sneakers for their mother who was incontinent and needed washable shoes. Another family brought in a cassette recorder with prerecorded tapes of family members' conversations and messages to their grandfather.

It is not necessary to have something in hand. Take him out for a drive or bring a picnic lunch to share on the patio. Bring in grandchildren, your relative's friends, or even his pets. These are enjoyable ways to show that you care and are thinking of him. If you think of the visit as a neighborly one, many ideas will come to mind.

Q: Is a resident's room ever changed even if he doesn't want a different room?

A: If a resident's physical and/or mental needs can no longer be met on the unit, a room change may be suggested. However, the resident (and a family member or legal representative of the resident) should be notified in advance of the transfer, unless contraindicated by a medical emergency that requires an immediate transfer. For instance, a resident who is diagnosed with an infection may have to be moved into a private room until he is found to be infection-free.

Discharge

Q: Why are some residents discharged?

A: There are several reasons. If a resident's condition improves, she may be moved to a less-structured environment, such as a group home. If she needs more skilled services than her facility is licensed and certified to provide, she may be transferred to another nursing home. For example, more intensive and skilled services may be required if she develops bedsores that need frequent treatment. She may then be discharged to a facility offering a higher level of care.

Discharge also occurs when a resident who has been on Medicare at the nursing home has fully recovered, is no longer eligible for Medicare skilled nursing home payment, and is ready to go home.

Some residents are discharged because they cause harm or are a threat to themselves or others. When this occurs, the doctor is notified and he gives the discharge order. The resident can either be sent to an acute hospital psychiatric unit for additional monitoring or be discharged home to his family. In cases where there is no family and the resident is incompetent, the Division of Elder Affairs can be notified and it, in turn, may act as the family representative to protect the rights of the resident.

Finally, there are times when family members are not satisfied with the nursing center for various reasons and decide to have their relative transferred to another facility.

They might have had unfortunate experiences with the original nursing home's staff or have been unhappy with the care their relative received. Also, families may have heard negative reports about their relative's nursing home and decided on a discharge.

Q: Can I take my relative out of the nursing home without the doctor's order?

A: A discharge should not take place without a physician's order. If a family member takes a resident home without a doctor's order, it is called a "discharge against medical advice." In such cases, the physician, as well as the nursing home, is legally cleared of any wrongdoing and is no longer responsible for the resident's welfare.

I strongly discourage you from taking this action, for several reasons. It can be very difficult to find a physician who will take over the care of your relative once he is aware that you have signed out against medical advice. Also, some insurance companies will not pay portions of the bill when this situation has occurred. Considering the high cost of nursing homes, it would be wise to check your insurance coverage concerning this.

If you are strongly considering taking this action, talk to the director of nurses and administrator and get another physician's opinion before moving your relative.

Q: How is a discharge handled?

A: There are several things you can expect on discharge day. First, if your relative is being transferred to another facility, in or out of the state, the charge nurse should provide all the necessary paperwork, copies of medical records, physician's orders, and a list of all the medications that your relative has been taking (including ones already taken that day). The nurse should also fill out a transfer record and check your relative to be sure she is in good physical condition before the discharge.

Next, he should help your relative pack her belongings, checking each item against the nursing home's record sheet; date and sign the personal item record; and ask you to do the same. This becomes your receipt for your relative's personal belongings. After that, he should take your relative to say goodbye to her friends, then take her to the front door, where the person in charge of transportation will take over. Later, the nurse will close out your relative's chart and ask the physician to write a summary discharge note on her medical record.

Finally, before you leave, the administrative department will give you a current itemized bill, any money or jewelry your relative left in the nursing home's safe, and a list of community services (if your relative is going home). No matter what the reason for discharge, everyone on the nursing home staff should offer you and your relative support on this last day.

In this chapter we have explored the answers to some frequently asked questions. In Chapter 7, you will learn how to recognize and effectively handle a variety of everyday problems.

7

Handling Problems

When your relative enters a nursing home, you have a new role to take on: you become her advocate. You and she together should monitor the care she receives and make sure the quality of her life does not needlessly decline. In all but the best nursing homes, there may be times when things go wrong. Staff members may be rude; there may be subtle or obvious abuse; there may be intentional or unintentional neglect. If you are a strong advocate for your relative, you can work with staff members to improve her care and eliminate problems.

Some people see a problem and charge in to correct it. Many other people are reluctant to confront an authority figure, especially one who seems to have superior knowledge. That's one reason why some families accept whatever a nurse, doctor, or administrator says. Another reason is that some families fear reprisals if they complain to the person in charge of their loved one. Yet the consequences of not bringing up a problem can be far worse than the consequences of speaking out to nursing home staff members.

Mrs. V.'s daughter was concerned about her mother's complaints of ridicule by a nurse. Her daughter would listen to these complaints but was afraid to talk with the nurse because she felt the staff might "take it out" on her mother. As time went on, Mrs. V. became increasingly depressed and even refused to go to activities. One day, Mrs. V.'s daughter came to visit and was told her mother was downstairs at a movie. This surprised her, since Mrs. V. had not been attending any programs. The next time she visited, her mother was out on the patio talking with other residents. When her daughter asked the nursing assistant about the change in her mother's

*moods and activities, she was told that a new nurse was
in charge of the unit. When she asked, her mother said
"I kept telling you how upset I was by her and you
would never listen. I was afraid to say anything to
anyone else and so I just didn't leave my room. She's
gone now and everyone else treats me so nice."*

Mrs. V. was extremely upset by one person on the staff, yet
both she and her daughter were afraid to confront the nurse
or talk to anyone about the problem.

If you are unhappy with the care your relative is receiving,
you should try to make the situation better. Nursing homes
that are concerned with a resident's welfare will welcome
your observations (and criticisms), and a nursing home that
doesn't is one in which you have to be especially watchful
and forceful in your job as advocate. Don't be intimidated.
If you present your concerns clearly, firmly, and persis-
tently, in a non-threatening way, you can truly affect the
care your relative receives.

In this chapter, I will tell you what to watch for and how
to evaluate your relative's care; some kinds of abuse and
neglect are obvious, but others are not. I will also tell you
about problems you and your relative might encounter with
staff members or your relative's private physician. Finally,
I will show you where to turn for help and how to handle
your relative's problems effectively.

Abuse and Inadequate Care

Abuse, either physical or psychological, often goes hand
in hand with neglect and inadequate care. For instance, if a
resident is left to bathe on her own and is either refused help
or is spoken to in a rude, insolent manner when she asks
for assistance, she is being neglected and abused. If a
resident is transferred from her bed to a chair in a rough
manner and later is found with bruises, she has been
abused. A resident left sitting in excreta is an example of
serious neglect. If she is found with her wrists red from the
tension of a restraint left on too long, she has been physically abused as well as neglected.

Mental abuse is any situation that causes a resident to feel
an unnecessarily high level of fear, anxiety, agitation,
withdrawal, or other emotional distress. Mrs. V. was experiencing depression and anxiety because of the way one of the

nurses was treating her, and as a result began to withdraw from everyday activities. In another case, a resident was made to feel like a child for spilling food and was criticized in front of others. She was being abused. So was another resident when she was told to "Shut up and stop asking to go to the bathroom because I just took you five minutes ago." A female resident who was snuggled up in bed with her husband each morning was teased by the staff. Such ridicule also represents mental and emotional abuse.

As one can imagine, some cases of abuse are difficult to assess and validate. For instance, a resident reports that a nursing assistant has done something to cause him distress, but the person accused of the abuse presents a different description of the event. A resident's broken arm cannot always be traced to rough handling. Older residents with severe osteoporosis and brittle bones often develop pathological fractures (broken bones not due to injury). The bone fractures can occur during simple movements, such as changing position in bed. Some residents in terminal stages of a disease can develop pathological fractures, bruises, and skin discolorations. Therefore, it may be difficult to tell whether a swelling is caused by rough handling, disease, or a natural degeneration of the bones.

Broken bones and other physical injuries must be judged very carefully. Before a nurse or other authority decides whether an assistant is guilty of abuse, the nurse will want answers to these questions. Was the resident confused or alert? Are pathological fractures part of the resident's disease process or diagnosis? Who was responsible for the resident's care that morning? Has that nursing assistant had recent complaints made against her, been known to handle residents in a rough manner, or previously been reported for rudeness to patients? If so, she may well be guilty of abuse. However, if the resident suffers from severe arthritis or osteoporosis, if X-ray results in her chart show she has had previous fractures in the nursing home, the chances are she has suffered another pathological fracture and has not been a victim of abuse.

The doctor is always called when there are injuries. X-rays are taken (either at the facility or at a nearby hospital), and an incident report is filed by the nurse documenting the resident's complaint, the nursing assistant's response to the complaint, and the action taken. If physical abuse is witnessed by anyone or is immediately reported by the

resident when it occurs, the police are notified and an investigation is conducted. You should always be notified
immediately when any kind of accident or suspected abuse
occurs, even if there is no apparent injury at the time of the
accident.

*I was quite shocked when I visited my father and saw
a bruise over his eye. He was not able to tell me what
happened but the nurse looked at his chart and told me,
"He bumped into a door this morning." I reminded her
that someone should have notified me at the time of the
accident. She quickly apologized but said they had
forgotten to call since it was such a minor injury.*

That's one reason why it is important to leave emergency
phone numbers so you or other relatives can be reached
when an emergency arises.

Abuse may be particularly difficult to assess if your
relative is mentally impaired or disoriented. In one reported
incident of verbal abuse, a resident said that a nursing
assistant spoke rudely to her and made fun of her in front
of others. The nursing assistant reported that she was only
joking with the resident and laughing "with her, not at her."
The assistant said, "This resident is always accusing people
of laughing at her but she is very disoriented and gets situations and people mixed up!" All nurses have had this
experience and such cases are difficult to evaluate.

Abuse, neglect, and inadequate care can take many forms.
Some problems arise when routine procedures are not
followed. Mrs. B. reported that clean linens were not always
provided at the nursing home. The linens, contracted out to
a service, were not always delivered on time or were used
more quickly than they could be laundered and returned.
When this happened, hers and others' beds were made up
without blankets or with only one sheet. Yet, regulations tell
us that, for warmth and cleanliness, beds should always
have a bottom and a top sheet as well as a pillowcase,
blanket, and bedspread.

A more serious problem that can affect your relative is
theft. It is unfortunately true that some staff members
trusted with the care of nursing home residents steal from
them. This problem is rarely seen in facilities with full-time
staff charge nurses who know their employees well. If a

nurse suspects the theft of a resident's personal belongings, she will consult with both the director of nurses and the administrator to resolve the problem immediately.

Theft is more difficult to handle in nursing homes that do not have full-time staff nurses in charge but rather depend upon temporary nurses. In these nursing homes, nurses are not familiar with the staff and the residents, and cannot so easily identify who is stealing.

As with other forms of abuse and inadequate care, not all cases of theft are clean-cut. In one instance, the "theft" of a radio turned out to be a case of sharing and borrowing by residents. The resident who reported the radio missing had forgotten that she had lent it to another resident. The resident who borrowed the radio hadn't told anyone that she was taking it to her room. However, the resident who had borrowed the radio was known to the charge nurse as a chronic borrower, so the nurse checked with her first before reporting the item as having been stolen.

The Bluegrass Long-Term Care Ombudsman program in Kentucky can provide you with a brochure that suggests precautions you can take to prevent theft in the nursing home. The brochure also gives procedures to follow when you suspect that a theft has occurred. Write to: Bluegrass Long-Term Care Ombudsman Program, 1530 Nicholasville Rd., Lexington, Kentucky 40503.

If your relative complains about any aspect of her care, sort out what she tells you in light of what you know about her personality, alertness, and adjustment to life in the nursing home. If her reports seem at all plausible, you should follow up on them, using the techniques described later in this chapter.

Ms. C. told her family that every night a strange man would come in her room and wake her up. She was beginning to have trouble sleeping and was afraid to tell the nurse. After talking to the nurse, the family members found out that an orderly worked the night shift and did go into the residents' rooms every two hours to check on their safety. Since Ms. C. had never married, she was very upset by a strange man entering her room during the night. When the orderly's presence in her room was explained, she understood and began again to sleep during the night without fear.

Long-term care ombudsmen usually list complaints in categories. These categories may be nursing, dietary, physical environment, financial, medical, legal, and administrative problems. Not everyone will have complaints in all these categories, but it is not unusual that little things may go wrong with any of these services.

Problems with Staff Members

During my years in nursing homes, I've seen all kinds of staff members. Most, fortunately, have been compassionate, caring individuals; some have not. I'm going to tell you about the kinds of people—from administrators to nursing assistants—who can adversely affect your relative's quality of life. If staff members like these work in your relative's nursing home, you will have to monitor them carefully and be prepared to be a strong advocate for improved conditions.

The administrator greatly influences the atmosphere and quality of a nursing home. A concerned, involved administrator sets a positive example for her staff, but if the administrator is distant and careless, your relative's care may suffer.

Ms. M. had cared for the elderly as a nurse for several years and made the decision to become an administrator. On any given day, she could be found in her office behind closed doors, smoking one cigarette after another, moving reams of paperwork across her cluttered desk, and shouting orders to those around her. The nursing director found her unapproachable and insensitive to the residents' and employees' needs. At five o'clock each day, Ms. M. was out the door on her way home, leaving behind unanswered questions and unfinished work.

Ms. M. was very impressed with her new position, but no one was impressed with Ms. M.! Several months went by. One day federal surveyors were present during one of her frequent shouting matches with a resident. The surveyors questioned the residents about the staff's attitudes and learned that Ms. M. spoke to everyone in a curt, abrasive way, alienating employees, residents, and families. Weeks later, Ms. M. was replaced.

A very few administrators are not receptive to residents and lack the warmth and personal interest needed to have good relations with families and staff. Additionally, they may turn a deaf ear to the requests of the nursing staff, a situation that can result in chaos.

I know of one director of nurses who tried to make her administrator aware that a particular unit was overburdened. The administrator ignored her, and the staff became disgruntled; there was a shortage of help and supplies. Survey reports were poor and after two negative inspections the director of nurses resigned. The unit continued short-staffed, and eventually the nursing home lost its right to accept new admissions until corrections were made. Ultimately, the administrator made the changes, hired a new director of nurses, and slowly improved conditions. However, many residents suffered in the meantime because of the administrator's shortsightedness.

This is typical of what can happen when there is a breakdown in communications and working relationships, coupled with a loss of respect between departments. The director of nurses, who is experienced in nursing care needs, asks for help and offers suggestions to improve the quality of care. The administrator, due either to lack of respect for the nursing needs of the facility or to lack of experience in the nursing care of the elderly, chooses to disregard the director's suggestions, with traumatic results.

A difficult situation can also occur if she is unsuited for her position. If the director is a domineering authoritarian, the results can be disastrous, even resulting in the loss of human life. Be wary of the director of nurses who tells you that your loved one's agitation, pain, weight gain, increased confusion, insomnia, lack of appetite, or other physical discomfort is due to aging, crankiness, or too much or too little activity. Be prepared to ask for documentation from the doctor stating that, for example, "crankiness" is the reason for your relative's weight loss. It requires a nurse who is caring, empathetic, and concerned about the needs of the elderly to find the underlying causes of her residents' symptoms. A head nurse who trivializes or dismisses your relative's symptoms is not doing her job!

Your relative is under the direct care of a charge nurse. A

charge nurse who fails to provide the right information to her nursing assistants, does not get involved in hands-on patient care, and tends only to the administrative work of the unit may find that she has lost control of her staff. You will know when this happens because the nursing unit will appear disorganized and many residents will suffer from bedsores or other signs of inadequate attention. Such a nurse lacks the skills to provide high-quality care.

There are geriatric nurses who follow the same routine every day, offering no variety for residents. Families of these residents complain, "Poor Mother! She's been doing the same, boring thing for months!" Occasionally a family says that their relative sits in front of the television all day long. There is no reason for this condition.

The employees who spend the most time with nursing home residents are the nursing assistants. Occasionally you may find a nursing assistant who lacks compassion and is tactless, unreliable, loud, offensive in her speech and rough in the care she gives. She is emotionally upsetting to residents, family, and staff. You may wonder, why was she hired and why was her behavior not recognized before she was entrusted with the care of the elderly? The answer is, no test or technique can unfailingly identify which people in a nursing assistant training course are unsuited for work with the elderly. Undesirable personality traits can be hidden for periods of time, but eventually supervisors will recognize the unqualified nursing assistant and ask her to leave her position.

Nationwide, research projects are in progress, focusing on the question, "Can caring and nurturing attitudes be learned by caregivers as are other subjects?" Initial results indicate that caring attitudes can be *taught* but that compassion cannot be acquired through learning. Rather, compassion, or the lack of it, is part of the inherent makeup of a personality.

Undesirable employees, be they administrators, directors of nursing, charge nurses, or nursing assistants, do not belong in nursing homes. Nevertheless, I've been in facilities where employees suspected of mental or physical abuse were allowed to continue working. I have read charts of residents who were victims of alleged abuse. Some of these alert residents actually named the nursing assistant involved and the person was still employed at the facility.

Mrs. C. would tell her family that she was not assisted with feeding, dressing, toileting, and was left to do everything for herself. She would ask for help in walking and the nursing assistant would not listen. If she asked for fresh water, she didn't get it. According to her doctor's orders, she was to be taken to the bathroom every two hours, and yet when the two hours was up and no one had taken her, the nurse would scold her for asking, when "We are too busy."

How can this happen? Some nursing home administrators and directors of nurses may hesitate to fire employees because they fear staff shortages. However, nursing homes should not compromise high-quality care because of such fear. Other administrators are afraid of litigation from terminated employees. Yet there are specific rules administrators can follow to avoid being sued. After all charges against an employee have been documented in written notices, and conferences between the administrator and offending employees have been documented, undesirable employees can and should be dismissed.

Questions about the Doctor

"I never get to talk with the doctor for more than five minutes and he's out the door!" or "He doesn't tell me what he's going to do, what tests he's ordering, or what medicines he's going to give me, he just does it. He seems to forget that I can still think."

These may be your relative's complaints. Some doctors are not trained to care for the aged and some are uncomfortable around elderly people. If you are dissatisfied with your relative's doctor, talk to her about his attitudes towards nursing home residents, and consider switching doctors if necessary.

Dr. L. was totally unfamiliar with the appropriate dosages of geriatric medications, apathetic towards nursing home patients, and unpleasant when the nurses approached her with their concerns. When Dr. L. failed to come for a scheduled visit, the medical director asked her to withdraw from a resident's case. She agreed. She was not emotionally prepared for the problems of the elderly and therefore did not provide quality care.

The private physician's responsibility, after the initial admissions examination, is to visit your relative at least every thirty days for the first ninety days, according to federal regulations. After that, the physician may see her patient less frequently if the nursing home's medical director approves.

If doctors don't visit residents according to the required schedule, the nursing home is considered "out of compliance" with the federal regulations and may lose its Medicare or Medicaid funding from the government. To avoid this, the nursing director will contact the medical director, who in turn will call the physician to remind her to visit or who will obtain the services of a physician to provide medical care as required. Sometimes, it is even necessary to ask the family to call the attending physician and remind her to visit the resident. A physician who is this inattentive is probably not giving her patient adequate care.

What to Do

You come to visit in the nursing home and the floor in your relative's room is dirty and there is an offensive odor. Your relative tells you that the room has not been cleaned in two days. You don't want to bother the nurse and you know that cleaning is not the nursing assistant's job. You go to the housekeeper on the floor and ask her about it.

You are more likely to get results when you discuss the problem with the responsible employee when you are dissatisfied with any aspect of your relative's care. You will be most effective if you state your concern in an objective, nonjudgmental way. If you verbally attack the employee or become very emotional, it is only natural that she will be defensive.

Here are some examples of how to approach employees successfully:

You find your relative without fresh drinking water close by. Ask her nurse for the name of the assistant in charge of your relative's care. Calmly ask the assistant to please keep fresh water available for your relative. Tell her you know she didn't intentionally forget the water, and that you understand how oversights happen.

As long as you give your request without emotion and blame, she should be very willing to do as you ask.

Another example:

You visit your mother and find that the wheelchair you gave her has the wrong footrests attached to it. This situation is not unusual. After you talk with the nursing assistants, go to the charge nurse and tell her: "I've found that labeling the items that belong together, such as the footrests to Mom's wheelchair, keeps parts from being misplaced. Maybe if you label these footrests along with her wheelchair, the correct footrests will always be put on the right chair. I can label them while I'm here if you'd like."

In this way, no one is blamed. Instead, you have made an objective observation and given a possible solution.

Perhaps you are concerned about your relative's sleeping habits. Tell the nurse your concerns.

"Whenever I visit Mother, she is always asleep. It's lunch time and she can barely stay awake long enough to eat her lunch. What do you think is the reason for this?"

If you present the problem this way, without blame, the nurse will be more inclined to discuss her observations about your mother's sleeping habits and the possible causes for her lunch-time naps. It may take a while to resolve the problem, but the nurse will keep you informed.

If you have a problem to discuss with the nurse, ask her to tell you which times during the day she is free to talk. There are hours that are more stressful than others in a nursing home, and the nurse will appreciate that you recognize the value of good timing. You will find the staff more willing to talk when they know you have waited for the right time to approach them.

You may not be able to resolve your problem by talking with nursing staff members; in that case, you should talk with the director of nurses. When you meet with her, vague references to problem areas won't be very helpful. You may find that keeping a log of incidents as they occur will enhance your memory and make you a more effective advocate for your relative.

The director of nurses should value your feedback about the charge nurses on your relative's unit. The feedback helps her determine how effective her charge staff is and where they should be placed. If you have good feelings about your relative's charge nurse, pass that on to the director; an honest compliment now may give your later questions and concerns more credibility. Also, if you feel that the director of nurses is a compassionate person who is always available to discuss your concerns, tell her so. Nursing home personnel like to know that they have contributed to the care and well-being of the residents and their families.

On the other hand, if after talking with the director of nurses, you are not pleased with her response and you feel that she is lacking in communication and nursing skills, ask for a conference with the administrator. Be as objective as possible. State your problems clearly and concisely and tell her the director of nurses' response to your concerns. If you know you will feel upset discussing nursing problems with the administrator, write the problems down ahead of time and read them to her. Another possibility is to send her a written complaint (see Appendix A).

Nursing homes offer another way to deal with problems: residents' councils which, among other things, meet to discuss grievances. Some councils are more effective than others, depending on the amount of encouragement shown by the nursing home's administrator. If your relative's home has an effective council, you can work with its members to resolve complaints. If the administrator tends to ignore the council's requests, ask the director of nurses and/or the social worker to attend a council meeting with you. Together, you may be able to get the administrator's attention.

It may happen that you can't solve your problem within the nursing home and have to turn to outside help. Organizations such as The National Citizens' Coalition for Nursing Home Reform offer support and advice. You can contact them at 1424 16th St., Suite L2, Washington, D.C. 20036.

Occasionally, residents or families may have complaints involving the administrator. Some of these complaints may be the attitude of the administrator, policies of the nursing home, lack of response to requests, extra charges for services which were not rendered, or lack of information on charges. The resident's council is helpful in solving many administrative problems that occur. If there is still a lack of response to complaints, the ombudsman should be notified.

Your local long-term care ombudsman investigates and resolves complaints about nursing homes, monitors state and federal laws affecting nursing homes, provides information to various agencies relating to long-term care issues, and trains staff and volunteers in the program. The long-term care ombudsman also has a wealth of information on local nursing homes. Contact your state's director on aging for information on the ombudsman's program in your area (see Appendix B).

The quality of a resident's life in a nursing home is the top priority of the ombudsmen. Turn to them for help with individual problems or for information about nursing home issues.

Your final option in the face of problems is to transfer your relative to another nursing home. This is a major step and one that should only be taken after a great deal of thought and discussion.

QUESTIONS TO ASK BEFORE LEAVING A NURSING HOME

• Are you pleased most of the time?
• Are your complaints shared by others?
• Have you tried to resolve your differences through every channel available?
• Has the nursing home been cited because of complaints?
• Does the problem undermine your relative's quality of life?

In your job as advocate, you have to weigh the answers to these questions carefully. Most problems can be resolved, but inadequate care may lead you, finally, to move on to another nursing home.

In Chapter 8, you will learn about the several stages of dying, ethical issues that occur in the nursing home, and how to comfort those who are terminally ill.

8

Dying in a Nursing Home

This book is about the quality of life, including the quality of the end of life. Many residents will spend their final days in nursing homes, and they will need the same attention and care then as they did during their first days in the nursing home. If you are like most people, you "put off thinking about death," says Dr. Robert N. Butler, the founding director of the National Institute of Aging. Perhaps the loss is too painful to contemplate or you feel helpless in the face of death. However, when it is time, there are things you can do to help your relative die in dignity and peace. You can make sure he is as comfortable as possible, you can surround him with love, you can help him accept his coming death, you can make it easier for him to say his good-byes, and you can let him know he is not alone.

In this chapter, I will help you understand the needs of the dying as explained in the classic book, *On Death and Dying*, by Dr. Elizabeth Kübler-Ross. I will also describe what happens in the nursing home when someone dies—who makes the phone calls, who takes care of the body. In addition, I have included a discussion of AIDS. As I write this book, there is no cure for this deadly disease, so patients with AIDS who come to a nursing home in the terminal stages of their illness have really come to die. Their special needs, and the quality of their life and dying, should be talked about.

In years past, relatives died at home in familiar surroundings. After the funeral, the home was filled with family and friends—grieving together, each person offered the others strength and support. Death was seen as an inevitable part of the natural order of things.

Compare this to the present-day dehumanizing process of dying in white-walled hospitals, surrounded by nurses and doctors draped in dull green cloth. Intravenous tubes, wires attached to monitors, respirators—all are hooked up, plugged in, and lit up. We well may wonder, "Is this what it's all about?"

Granted, everyone is thankful to have the marvels of science. Nonetheless, they all seem so foreign that you might feel a strange antagonism toward the entire process of dying in an institution, thinking it might be better to die peacefully at home.

When you think about death, you are probably struck with the reality of your relative's and your own vulnerability. Your emotions and the emotions of the dying person are very complex. Let the information in this chapter be a guide through this difficult time. It should help you talk to your relative about death and respond to him in comforting and compassionate ways.

AIDS

More and more, AIDS victims are entering nursing homes for care. AIDS is a devastating new viral disease characterized by the breakdown of the body's immune system. When this system is not working normally, recurrent infections set in and cause progressive weakness. Eventually he will die of complications due to his disease. Despite intensive research, a proven method of treatment for AIDS has not yet been discovered; however, there are many experimental drugs being used. Patients with this disease cannot live out their remaining days in a hospital, nor can they care for themselves as they become weaker. Families and friends have been known to turn their backs on an infected person. As the public learns more about this disease, much of the fear surrounding it will disappear. Until then, living arrangements present a major problem, and young patients with AIDS may find themselves faced with admission to a nursing home.

The states decide which nursing homes are qualified to receive Medicaid funds for the care of residents with AIDS. The nursing home administrators set the policies of their individual nursing homes. Before accepting AIDS patients, the administrator and the director of nurses must be sure their facility can provide both appropriate training and continued support for the staff members.

Nursing homes have a great deal of experience in caring

for residents with other viral infections including flu, shingles, and hepatitis. Much is known about these diseases and they are treatable; AIDS is different. However, with continuing education, nursing home staffs have become qualified to handle residents suffering from AIDS.

All levels of employees in a nursing home with AIDS residents are given in-depth education. The Centers for Disease Control recommends that the same routines and precautions be followed with AIDS patients that are already followed with hepatitis B patients. A patient with AIDS will have a private room or will share a room with another resident with AIDS. He shouldn't be confined to his room or be restricted from any activities, provided he has the strength to attend and participate.

The problems and concerns of the person dying of AIDS are different from those of the elderly. The AIDS resident may be hostile and resentful of his disease and the isolation forced on him by family and friends. It may be very difficult for him to accept himself and his diagnosis and he may feel extreme guilt, anger, frustration, and depression. If he is to find any peace, he needs a chance to vent his feelings without fear of recrimination. There are numerous groups and resource centers which offer support to AIDS victims and their families.

For information and referrals for psychological counseling, contact:

> American Psychological Association
> 1200 17th Street, N.W.
> Washington, D.C. 20036
> Attn: Dr. Jacquelyn Gentry

You can also contact:

> The AIDS Clearing House
> 1-800-458-5231
> (for information, resource materials,
> and referral services)

A good nursing home will try to meet the emotional, physical, and spiritual needs of an individual with AIDS. It is not enough to nurse him along physically; in the nursing home, he should find the highest quality of life possible for his remaining days.

The Stages of Dying

Dr. Elizabeth Kübler-Ross wrote a moving and illuminating book, *On Death and Dying.* In her book, she described the five stages that a terminally ill person goes through: *denial, anger, bargaining, depression,* and finally, *acceptance.* Not all people go through these stages in a clearly defined manner. Some may pass over one or two stages while others never do reach the *acceptance* stage.

We all tend to deny certain aspects of life, such as aging and illness. It is as though we seek refuge and find it in denial. We can look at others who are aging or ill and say, "Not me, thank God." When a person is faced with a terminal diagnosis, is it any wonder that he responds with denial? My father, when he learned of his terminal cancer, truly believed that if he stopped smoking, he might prolong his life. All of us have read of famous people who have gone to great lengths to receive all forms of "new treatments" in other countries, in hopes of warding off the inevitable. These are all methods of *denying* the facts.

Once a person gets through the denial stage, providing he has time, he will use less radical defense mechanisms. We cannot hope to change this process, nor should we try, since a dying person should be allowed to go through this denial stage, resolving it in the way most acceptable to him. We should instead help with his care and anticipate his needs. We must look for signs that he is ready to accept the inevitable, and we should prepare to be there for him when that time comes.

After the denial stage, when the dying patient begins to realize that he has an incurable disease, he feels *anger*: first, at the doctor who diagnosed him and then at himself, for his inability to control and cure the disease. He is angry that this has happened to him and not to the hundreds of "no-goods" who have brought only pain and suffering to others. "Why me?" He ponders this question night and day. Only through discussion, and perhaps counseling, can he begin to focus on the reality of his anger as a natural stage in the dying process. This stage can be the most difficult one for a resident's family, for at times he directs his hostility toward them. The staff also finds this a difficult stage since the resident now makes loud demands on them and may ring for them incessantly or give abrasive responses to their questions. It's as though he wants to remind the staff that he is still alive. At this time all the family and staff can do is to offer comfort.

In the next stage of dying, the resident begins to think that if he can figure out a way, he might be able to *bargain* for time and his life. "What if I give up all my material things, go to church every day, give my right arm to have my life, quit smoking two packs of cigarettes a day, maybe then—? Can I bargain in some way for this life and somehow postpone the inevitable?" When he realizes this can't be done, the individual comes closer to the final stage of *acceptance*. Before the acceptance occurs, however, he may become extremely *depressed*.

There are so many things in life to be done, so many amends to be made (and indeed he should be allowed to make them), so much he wants to see, so many places to go, projects to finish, grandchildren, yet unborn, to hold and love, and children and family to provide for. How can he leave now? Who will pay the bills? He thinks of all these things, even dreams of them. He feels a deep sense of loss. We must remember, above all, not to prolong his depression by offering false support or sunny thoughts. It may be necessary for the nursing staff to provide sedation at this point, along with pain medication, to alleviate physical or mental discomfort. He has come to the final stage.

During the course of a terminal illness the stages of dying may not always be clearly defined and a resident may go in and out of these stages several times before death occurs. Many ethical and moral problems may arise that, if handled with understanding and sensitivity, can add dignity and quality to your loved ones's remaining days.

The following story is an example of how the staff of one nursing home helped a resident in his search for quality of life during his terminal illness.

Mr. T., a very alert and oriented seventy-nine-year-old man, was admitted to the nursing home for rehabilitation and physical therapy after bilateral hip replacements for degenerative arthritis. Months prior to the surgery, he had been diagnosed as having prostate cancer, which had now spread to his bones but had not been causing Mr. T. any pain up to this time.

Mr. T.'s first quality-of-life decision was whether to have surgery on his hips when his cancer had already spread to the bones. After much discussion with his doctor and wife, Mr. T. decided he would rather have surgery and spend his remaining days walking than to be incapacitated in functioning because of degenerative arthritis in his hips.

In the nursing home, Mr. T. did well in physical therapy and regaining strength until he began having pain in his shoulders and spine. Bone scans now showed cancer in these new areas. This new development was discussed with Mr. T. and again, after talking with his wife, he agreed on a course of radiation and then chemotherapy. After several weeks of severe side effects from the therapies, Mr. T. began refusing treatments.

The doctor had told Mr. T. there was a very low probability that chemotherapy or further radiation would make any difference in his prognosis. Mr. T. then had to consider what quality his life would have if he continued with therapy or if he refused treatments.

Mr. T.'s doctor tried to convince him to continue with chemotherapy but Mr. T. said he wanted to make the decision for himself.

After consideration and discussion with his doctor, clergy, and family, Mr. T. declined further treatment and asked to be kept as comfortable and pain-free as possible. He began to take an injectable pain medication when he needed it. But the medication caused him to suffer severe side effects: confusion and an increasing loss of balance that resulted in several falls. After a few days, an oral pain medicine was started, but again Mr. T. suffered side effects. He became constipated and despite laxatives, now required daily enemas.

After weeks of pain medicine, laxatives, and enemas, Mr. T. one day called in the nurse and doctor. He said he was very depressed and did not want to continue with the painful enemas every day nor did he feel there was any meaning left to his life. He had accomplished the feat of walking after his surgery, he had no regrets for having gone through with it, but he did not want to go on like this. He asked to stop the enemas. The doctor and nurse explained that the enemas were preventing a bowel obstruction, of which Mr. T. was already aware. He declined further treatment and said he wanted to be left alone, even if his death was imminent.

Mr. T. is just one of many alert, intelligent, and coherent residents in nursing homes who daily face quality-of-life decisions, not just once, but several times during the course of an illness. These decisions are difficult, not only for the resident who must make the choices, but for his family and the nursing home staff.

Mr. T. came to *accept* the fact that he had an incurable illness, was *angry* about it, but could not *bargain* it away, and naturally was *depressed* by his loss of control over the illness. Once he accepted that his condition was beyond his power to change, that life goes on, even into another lifetime (if so he believed), and that the end was near, he was ready to enter the last stage of his life.

It is important to remember that as long as your loved one is competent and able to make his own decisions, his choices should be respected and he should be supported during these times by family, support groups, clergy or rabbi, and the nursing home's social worker. He should not be made to feel guilty if he decides something in his best interest but not necessarily yours.

You can help your loved one maintain a control over his life as well as his impending death, to the best of his ability, by respecting his wishes and thereby ensuring a sense of dignity to the dying process.

The family may need a great deal of support during such a time, for a resident near the end of his life is tired and wants to be left alone to prepare for his death. Some family members actually take this display of listlessness and withdrawal as a form of rejection by the dying loved one. They may try in vain to get him to "hang on" and not leave them. This is extremely cruel to the person who has reached this point and is now preparing in the way that he knows best.

In my years of nursing, I have found that by the time a resident reaches this stage, he is no longer afraid of death, but welcomes it. I have heard a resident say, "Don't be afraid for me—be thankful that I will be in peace and without suffering. It has been a long, hard struggle to get to this point." He should be allowed all the peace and quiet he needs.

Friends, relatives, volunteers, or employees at the nursing home can help the dying resident carry the burden he must bear and provide an outlet for any anger, fear, and hostility he feels along the way. If your relative is dying, you can arrange for him to see clergy or visit with friends to whom

he wishes to make amends. He may express himself as he
never has before. Allow him to talk of the past, the good as
well as the bad, recalling memories of his youth and his
family life. You can sit with him, read, pray (if this is his
request), hold his hand, and comfort him.

Always remember that even if you suspect he becomes
unconscious and unaware of his surroundings, you can
never be sure. Always treat him as though he were alert and
aware and try to say something calming, for it is suggested
that hearing may be the last sense to leave the body. A
study conducted at the Hartford Hospital in Connecticut tells
us that more may occur in the unconscious than what we
suspect. It may even be that feelings and even sights, as well
as sounds, are a part of the unconscious world. Since no one
knows what he is experiencing, every effort must be made
to respect his senses. Always remember this when visiting
comatose, or semi-comatose patients. They may not see and
speak—but they do hear!

Try to anticipate his needs, physical and emotional, and
provide for him. You may have to be extremely perceptive
and watch for signs of his needs. This may be very difficult
for you, especially if there is no response. You may see
worry lines on his face, his fists clenched, an agitated
restlessness, or you may see no visible signs of discomfort
at all. You may even have to ask questions, "Do you need
a pain shot?" or "Do you want me closer to you?" or "Do
you want a cool cloth on your forehead?" The staff may
assist you in finding out if he needs anything. The most
important thing is to be there with him if at all possible.
Just your presence at the bedside can allay his worst fears.
Don't be afraid of physical contact. Chances are that this is
what he needs most.

*Every nurse remembers her first dying patient and
when I was taking care of Bob, a nineteen-year-old, I felt
the life leaving his body as I held him and talked to him.
He had been unresponsive for days and the doctors said
he did not recognize anyone now and felt no pain. Yet,
just before he died, his eyes turned to look at me as I
took care of him, and as I spoke and moved around, his
eyes followed me. I was certain that he knew me as the
nurse who had taken care of him for the past several
weeks and I felt that he heard me as I talked to him in
those last few hours.*

Your relative may ask to leave his body to research or donate his organs. Respect his wishes and do all in your power to follow his requests. If he wishes to draw up a living will during this stage, honor the request.

When his time is near, allow him to die peacefully. There is nothing more upsetting than to hear relatives present at the bedside of a dying person crying, "Please don't leave us, Dad," or "I can't live without you." Rather, say, "I love you and I'm here with you—here is my hand." Allow your relative to die in a quiet, dignified way. This much respect we all owe to life and to the dying.

When Death Occurs

When a resident dies in a nursing home, the staff, the family, and the other residents all have strong feelings they must deal with. There are practical matters to be dealt with, too. This section will tell you what happens right after a death.

If the resident's death was sudden, his charge nurse will call the family and the resident's doctor, who will come to the nursing home to sign the death certificate. If the doctor has not seen the resident recently, the local coroner's office will also be called to conduct an investigation of the death. In addition, the nurse or the family will call the funeral home and the nurse will contact any organizations to which the resident has donated his organs.

The family, if it wants, may have a final visit before the resident's body is transferred to the funeral home. The staff will make sure the resident's door is kept closed and that the family has privacy. When the funeral director arrives, he will be escorted quietly and quickly to the room, and other residents will be kept out of the area until he is finished.

The nurses will pack the deceased resident's personal belongings and sign the necessary release forms. If the resident had a roommate, that person may be having a difficult time accepting the death of his friend and may need light sedation.

There is no easy way to deal with dying—this is true even with the elderly who have lived full lives—and there are many quality-of-life issues to be dealt with even at this time. Everyone is upset at the time of death and the residents are very aware of when a death occurs. The only consolation for them, the staff, and the family during this time may come from acknowledging their feelings of loss and sadness and knowing that the love and care the dying resident received added to the quality of his life during his final days.

Afterword

Working for Change

On your own, you can make significant improvements in the quality of care and the quality of life your relative has in the nursing home. As part of a citizens' group, you can help change the way all nursing home residents are treated. National and community organizations are actively working on many fronts—Congress, city hall, and nursing home offices—to improve long-term care for the elderly. You can help by letting government officials know you care about the quality of life in nursing homes and getting involved in an advocacy group. Additionally, you must be willing to support increased funding to pay for needed care as the population ages and care needs become more complex.

Government Action

The U.S. Congress has long been involved in regulating nursing homes to ensure the highest quality care possible. Recent congressional action has been aimed at preventing discrimination against low-income nursing home residents, improving special training for nursing staffs, and requiring detailed background pre-employment checks on direct caregivers.

New bills have placed more emphasis on residents' rights. In late 1987, Congress passed a law strengthening the Long-Term Care Ombudsman program. Under Public Law 100-175, states must give ombudsmen more power and greater access to nursing homes and official records. This means that ombudsmen, the official advocates for residents, will be in a better position to improve conditions in nursing homes. New legislation has also proposed improvements in the inspections of nursing homes, and penalties for nursing

135

homes that retaliate against residents who complain about conditions.

Congress frequently considers bills to improve the regulation and quality of our nation's nursing homes. If you are interested in current legislation, call (202) 224-3121 and ask the U.S. Capitol operator to connect you with your congressman or congresswoman's office. A staffer there can put you in touch with whoever is working on nursing home issues.

Citizen Involvement

Until recently, the medical field generally felt immune to the criticisms of the public. Whatever decisions a doctor or other members of a medical institution made, whether quality of life was affected or not, became law. Doctors and nursing home administrators were the "professionals" entrusted with the care of loved ones and were respected for that fact alone.

Public organizations, advocacy groups, and attention to the motivation of nursing home management and staff have changed all that and greatly influenced the care given in medical settings. Complacency and apathy have never brought about changes in nursing homes; only action and involvement have led to improvements.

Most nursing homes now provide at least adequate care. Nevertheless, facts and figures supplied by the Special Committee on Aging and the reports of national ombudsmen and citizens' advocacy groups cannot be taken lightly. There are still many problems. A 1984 states' ombudsmen report cited the need for improved nursing home regulations, better staff training, more staff to care for residents, and better pay for nursing assistants. The report also gave examples of inadequate care in some of the nation's nursing homes: poor hygiene, lost items, unanswered calls for help, negative staff attitudes, abuse, and neglect.

The National Citizens' Coalition for Nursing Home Reform (NCCNHR) has embarked on a national campaign to increase public awareness of nursing home issues. Members of congress and prominent Americans endorsed the NCCNHR's efforts and called for support of regulatory reforms. The Institute of Medicine's report, "Improving the Quality of Care in Nursing Homes," indicated that "profound regulatory changes" must take place. Many changes have taken effect since this report, and conditions in the nation's nursing homes are improving, but it will require ongoing effort and hard work on everyone's part to ensure that the improvement continues.

Consumers today are better educated and have a right to know why certain nursing homes are permitted to operate after violating a federal requirement, or why some facilities that are known to be substandard are allowed to operate and receive federal funds. If a nursing home's conditions fall below federal standards, concerned citizens want to know what corrective actions they can take. Families of elderly relatives are eager to become involved in citizens' groups for the betterment of nursing homes. They want to know about current and pending legislation that will ensure high-quality nursing home care.

Resource centers, including the NCCNHR, the Administration on Aging, state divisions of licensing and certification of nursing homes, and the Long-Term Care Ombudsman Program are vast libraries of information on nursing home care. If you want to work for nursing home reform, any of these organizations can put you in touch with local groups.

Praise should go to all who are concerned with our aging population. They find the time to become involved in improving the elderly's quality of life. One day, through their good efforts, there may be excellent nursing home care for all who need it.

Appendix A

A Resident's Bill of Rights

A resident's Bill of Rights is a declaration pertaining to the safety, well-being, and privacy of each resident in a nursing home. In some states provisions mandating the residents' rights may be found in the licensing and certification regulations. Proven violation of these rights can result in legal action against the facility for inappropriate care of its residents. The list of rights is posted in facilities in several places so you may refer to it as the need arises. The full resident's rights bill is quite lengthy. What follows is a general overview of these rights:

- Every resident shall be treated with respect and full recognition of her dignity and individuality.
- Every resident, prior to or at the time of admission, shall receive a written statement of the provided services at the facility and those that require extra charge (inclusive of Medicare or Medicaid non-covered services).
- Every resident shall receive complete and current information concerning her health and medical condition, in terms she can understand, from her physician, unless the physician decides that informing the resident is medically contraindicated. She will participate in the planning of this treatment or may refuse medication and treatment.
- Every resident shall be given privacy and respect during treatment and care of personal needs.
- Every resident's medical record shall be treated in confidence, and the written consent of the resident or family shall be obtained to release the records to any individual not otherwise authorized to receive it, except as needed in the case of the resident's transfer to another health care facility or as required by law or third-party payment contract.
- Every resident shall be free from mental and physical abuse and free from chemical and physical restraints except as authorized by a physician.
- Every resident shall be encouraged to submit complaints and recommendations concerning the nursing home's policies and

services to the staff or outside representatives of the resident's choice, or both. Such complaints shall be submitted free from restraint, coercion, discrimination, or reprisal.

- Every resident shall be informed of the relationship of this nursing home to any other health care facility insofar as the resident's care is concerned.
- Every resident shall be free to associate with persons and groups of her own choice unless this infringes upon another resident's rights.
- Every resident shall be assured of sending and receiving unopened personal mail.
- Every resident shall have the right to manage her financial affairs and may inspect her accounts and statements.
- Every resident shall have the right to retain her personal possessions and clothing, as space permits.
- Every resident shall have the right to remain in the facility and shall not be transferred or discharged, nor have her treatment altered radically, without prior consultation with the resident or, if the resident is incompetent, without prior notification of the next of kin or sponsor.
- Every married couple shall be afforded the right to privacy during their visits and, if both are residents of the facility, shall be offered the opportunity to share a room, unless medically contraindicated.
- Every resident shall have the opportunity to perform services for her own benefit and not for the sole benefit of the facility.
- The administrator shall be responsible for the implementations of all the residents' rights.
- The facility shall train the staff in the implementation of the residents' rights.

In addition to the residents' bill of rights, an admission agreement from the individual nursing home will be provided to you. While a resident is protected by her bill of rights, there may be some areas that are unclear in this bill but more succinct in an admission agreement. An example of one admission agreement is the resident's and the guarantor's acknowledgment that no person shall, without prior permission of the facility's administration, bring in food, medications, liquids, or smoking materials. The facility operates under the terms of Title VI of the Civil Rights Act of 1964 and thereby admits residents of any race, color, or national origin. Any infringements or complaints pertaining to the residents' Bill of Rights should be addressed to the State Office on Aging (see Appendix B) and to the Department of Licensing and Certification (see Appendix C).

Example of Complaint Procedure

The residents' Bill of Rights states that she has a right to present grievances and recommend changes to nursing home policies without the fear of recrimination. What is the procedure to be followed by the resident who has a complaint?

One facility's policies state that the following steps are to be followed:

- Make the effort to resolve the situation through the head of the department
- If a satisfactory conclusion is not possible, refer to the administrator, and she will work with the resident or the resident's agent in resolving the issue within four working days
- If the problem is unresolved at this level, the complaint is to be submitted to the executive committee, who will respond within ten working days
- If no conclusion can be reached and the problem is unresolved, a copy of the complaint and the response are to be forwarded to the State Office on Aging and the Department of Licensing and Certification

A complaint does not require signing by the resident or his family, but may be submitted by telephone, mail, office visits, or direct staff input.

Appendix B

Directory of State Agencies on Aging

ALABAMA
Dr. Oscar D. Tucker,
Executive Director
Alabama Commission on
Aging
136 Catoma Street, Second
Floor
Montgomery, AL 36130
205-261-5743

ALASKA
Ms. Connie Sipe, Executive
Director
Older Alaskans Commission
P.O. Box C, MS 0209
Juneau, AK 99811
907-465-3250

AMERICAN SAMOA
Mr. Sunuitao T. Tupai,
Director
Territorial Administration on
Aging
Government of American
Samoa
Pago Pago, AS 96799
684-633-1251

ARIZONA
Mr. Richard Littler,
Administrator
Aging and Adult
Administration
Department of Economic
Security
1400 West Washington Street
Phoenix, AZ 85007
602-542-4446
*1-800-352-3792

ARKANSAS
Mr. Herb Sanderson, Deputy
Director
Division of Aging and Adult
Services
Arkansas Department of
Human Services
Main and Seventh Streets
Donaghey Building, Suite
1428
Little Rock, AR 72201
501-682-2441

CALIFORNIA
Ms. Alice Gonzales, Director
California Department of
Aging
1600 K Street
Sacramento, CA 95814
916-322-5290

*In-State Toll-Free Number

141

COLORADO

Ms. Rita Barreras, Acting
  Director
Aging and Adult Services
Department of Social Services
1575 Sherman Street, Tenth
  Floor
Denver, CO 80203-1714
303-866-5905

COMMONWEALTH
OF THE NORTHERN
MARIANA ISLANDS

Mr. John Guerrero,
  Administrator
Office on Aging
Department of Community
  and Cultural Affairs
Civic Center
Commonwealth of the
  Northern Mariana Islands
Saipan, Mariana Islands
  96950
670-234-6011

CONNECTICUT

Ms. Mary Ellen Klinck,
  Commissioner
Connecticut Department on
  Aging
175 Main Street
Hartford, CT 06106
203-566-3238
*1-800-443-9946

DELAWARE

Ms. Eleanor L. Cain, Director
Delaware Division on Aging
Department of Health and
  Social Services
1901 North Dupont Highway,
  Second Floor
New Castle, DE 19720
302-421-6791
*1-800-223-9074

*In-State Toll-Free Number

DISTRICT OF COLUMBIA

Ms. E. Veronica Pace,
  Executive Director
District of Columbia Office on
  Aging
Executive Office of the Mayor
1424 K Street, NW, Second
  Floor
Washington, DC 20005
202-724-5622

FEDERATED STATES OF
MICRONESIA

Mr. Wehns Billen, Director
State Agency on Aging
Office of Health Services
Department of Social Services
Kolonia, Ponape,
Eastern Carolina Islands
  96941

FLORIDA

Dr. Larry Polivka
Assistant Secretary
Aging and Adult Services
Department of Health and
  Rehabilitative Services
Building 2, Room 328
1323 Winewood Boulevard
Tallahassee, FL 32399-0700
904-488-8922
*1-800-342-0825

GEORGIA

Mr. Fred McGinnis, Director
Office of Aging
Department of Human
  Resources, Sixth Floor
878 Peachtree Street, NE
Atlanta, GA 30309
404-894-5333

GUAM

Ms. Florence Shimizu,
Director
Division of Senior Citizens
Department of Public Health
and Social Services
P.O. Box 2816
Government of Guam
Agana, GU 96910
671-734-2942

HAWAII

Dr. Jeanette Takamura,
Executive Director
Hawaii Executive Office on
Aging
335 Merchant Street, Room
241
Honolulu, HI 96813
808-548-2593

IDAHO

Ms. Charlene W. Martindale,
Director
Idaho Office on Aging
Statehouse, Room 108
Boise, ID 83720
208-334-3833

ILLINOIS

Mrs. Janet S. Otwell, Director
Illinois Department on Aging
421 East Capitol Avenue
Springfield, IL 62701
217-785-2870
*1-800-252-8966

INDIANA

Mr. Barry A. Chambers,
Commissioner
Indiana Department of Human
Services
251 North Illinois Street
P.O. Box 7083
Indianapolis, IN 46207-7083
317-232-1139
*1-800-545-7763

*In-State Toll-Free Number

IOWA

Ms. Betty L. Grandquist,
Executive Director
Department of Elder Affairs
Jewett Building, Suite 236
914 Grand Avenue
Des Moines, IA 50319
515-281-5187
*1-800-532-3213

KANSAS

Ms. Esther Valladolid Wolf,
Secretary
Kansas Department on Aging
Docking State Office Building,
122-S
915 SW Harrison
Topeka, KS 66612-1500
913-296-4986
*1-800-432-3535

KENTUCKY

Mrs. Sue Tuttle, Director
Division for Aging Services
Cabinet for Human Resources
Department for Social Services
275 East Main Street
Frankfort, KY 40621
502-564-6930

LOUISIANA

Ms. Vicky Hunt, Director
Governor's Office of Elderly
Affairs
P.O. Box 80374
Baton Rouge, LA 70898-0374
504-925-1700

MAINE

Ms. Christine Gianopoulos,
Director
Bureau of Maine's Elderly
Department of Human
Services
State House, Station 11
Augusta, ME 04333
207-289-2561

MARYLAND

Mrs. Rosalie S. Abrams,
   Director
Maryland Office on Aging
301 West Preston Street
Baltimore, MD 21201
301-225-1102
*1-800-338-0153

MASSACHUSETTS

Mr. Paul J. Lanzikos,
   Secretary
Massachusetts Executive
   Office of Elder Affairs
38 Chauncy Street
Boston, MA 02111
617-727-7750
*1-800-882-2003

MICHIGAN

Ms. Olivia P. Maynard,
   Director
Office of Services to the Aging
P.O. Box 30026
Lansing, MI 48909
517-373-8230

MINNESOTA

Mr. Gerald A. Bloedow,
   Executive Secretary
Minnesota Board on Aging
Human Services Building,
   Fourth Floor
444 Lafayette Road
St. Paul, MN 55155-3843
612-296-2770
*1-800-652-9747

MISSISSIPPI

Dr. David K. Brown,
   Executive Director
Mississippi Council on Aging
301 West Pearl Street
Jackson, MS 39203-3092
601-949-2070
*1-800-222-7622

MISSOURI

Mr. Edwin Walker, Director
Division of Aging
Department of Social Services
2701 West Main Street
P.O. Box 1337
Jefferson City, MO 65102
314-751-3082
*1-800-235-5503

MONTANA

Mr. Robert L. Mullen, Director
Department of Family
   Services
P.O. Box 8005
Helena, MT 59604
406-444-5900
*1-800-332-2272

NEBRASKA

Ms. Betsy Palmer, Director
Department on Aging
301 Centennial Mall South
P.O. Box 95044
Lincoln, NE 68509
402-471-2306

NEVADA

Mrs. Suzanne Ernst,
   Administrator
Division for Aging Services
State Mail Room
Las Vegas, NV 89158
702-486-3545

NEW HAMPSHIRE

Mr. Richard A. Chevrefils,
   Director
Division of Elderly and Adult
   Services
New Hampshire Department
   of Health and Human
   Services
6 Hazen Drive
Concord, NH 03301
603-271-4390
*1-800-852-3311

*In-State Toll-Free Number

NEW JERSEY
Mrs. Ann Zahora, Director
New Jersey Division on Aging
Department of Community
  Affairs
101 South Broad Street, CN
  807
Trenton, NJ 08625-0807
609-292-0920
*1-800-792-8820

NEW MEXICO
Dr. Stephanie FallCreek,
  Director
New Mexico State Agency on
  Aging
La Villa Rivera Building,
  Fourth Floor
224 East Palace Avenue
Santa Fe, NM 87501
505-827-7640
*1-800-432-2080

NEW YORK
Mrs. Jane Gould, Director
New York State Office for the
  Aging
Agency Building #2
Empire State Plaza
Albany, NY 12223-0001
518-474-5731
*1-800-342-9871

NORTH CAROLINA
Mr. Alfred "Al" B. Boyles,
  Director
North Carolina Division of
  Aging
Department of Human
  Resources
Kirby Building, 1985 Umstead
  Drive
Raleigh, NC 27603
919-733-3983
*1-800-662-7030

NORTH DAKOTA
Larry Brewster, D.S.W.,
  Director
Aging Services Division
North Dakota Department of
  Human Services
State Capitol Building
Bismarck, ND 58505
701-224-2577
*1-800-472-2622

OHIO
Dr. Carol D. Austin, Director
Ohio Department of Aging
50 West Broad Street, Ninth
  Floor
Columbus, OH 43215
614-466-5500

OKLAHOMA
Mr. Roy R. Keen, Division
  Administrator
Aging Services Division
Department of Human
  Services
P.O. Box 25352
Oklahoma City, OK 73125
405-521-2327

OREGON
Mr. Richard C. Ladd,
  Administrator
Senior Services Division
Department of Human
  Resources
313 Public Service Building
Salem, OR 97310
503-378-4728

*In-State Toll-Free Number

PENNSYLVANIA

Dr. Linda M. Rhodes,
    Secretary
Pennsylvania Department of
    Aging
231 State Street (Barto
    Building)
Harrisburg, PA 17101
717-783-1550

PUERTO RICO

Dr. Celia Cintron, Executive
    Director
Puerto Rico Office of Elderly
    Affairs
Call Box 50063
Old San Juan Station, PR
    00902
809-721-0753

REPUBLIC OF THE MARSHALL ISLANDS

Mr. Winjang Ritok, Director
State Agency on Aging
Department of Social Services
Republic of the Marshall
    Islands
Marjuro, Marshall Islands
    96960

REPUBLIC OF PALAU

Ms. Lillian Nakamura,
    Director
State Agency on Aging
Department of Social Services
Republic of Palau
Koror, Palau 96940

RHODE ISLAND

Mrs. Adelaide Luber, Director
Department of Elderly Affairs
79 Washington Street
Providence, RI 02903
401-277-2858
*1-800-752-8088

SOUTH CAROLINA

Mrs. Ruth Q. Seigler,
    Executive Director
South Carolina Commission
    on Aging
400 Arbor Lake Drive, Suite
    B-500
Columbia, SC 29223
803-735-0210
*1-800-922-1107

SOUTH DAKOTA

Ms. Gail M. Ferris,
    Administrator
Office of Adult Services and
    Aging
Richard F. Kneip Building
700 Governors Drive
Pierre, SD 57501-2291
605-773-3656

TENNESSEE

Mrs. Emily M. Wiseman,
    Executive Director
Tennessee Commission on
    Aging
706 Church Street, Suite 201
Nashville, TN 37219-5573
615-741-2056

TEXAS

Mr. O. P. "Bob" Bobbitt,
    Executive Director
Texas Department on Aging
P.O. Box 12786, Capitol
    Station
Austin, TX 78711
512-444-2727
*1-800-252-9240

*In-State Toll-Free Number

UTAH

Mr. Percy Devine, III, Director
Utah Division of Aging and
  Adult Services
120 North 200 West, Room
  4A
P.O. Box 45500
Salt Lake City, UT 84145-
  0500
801-538-3910

VERMONT

Mr. Joel D. Cook,
  Commissioner
Department of Rehabilitation
  and Aging
103 South Main Street
Waterbury, VT 05676
802-241-2400
*1-800-642-5119

VIRGIN ISLANDS

Mrs. Juel C. Rhymer Molloy,
  Commissioner
Virgin Islands Department of
  Human Services
Barbel Plaza South
Charlotte Amalie
St. Thomas, VI 00802
809-774-0930

VIRGINIA

Ms. Wilda M. Ferguson,
  Commissioner
Virginia Department for the
  Aging
700 East Franklin Street,
  Tenth Floor
Richmond, VA 23219-2327
804-225-2271
*1-800-552-4464

*In-State Toll-Free Number

WASHINGTON

Mr. Charles E. Reed, Assistant
  Secretary
Aging and Adult Services
  Administration
Department of Social and
  Health Services
Mail Stop OB-44-A
Olympia, WA 98504
206-586-3768
*1-800-422-3263

WASHINGTON, D.C.

Administration on Aging
Office of State and Tribal
  Programs
Room 4752
330 Independence Avenue,
  S.W.
Washington, D.C. 20201

WEST VIRGINIA

Ms. Susan M. Harman,
  Executive Director
West Virginia Commission on
  Aging
State Capitol Complex, Holly
  Grove
1710 Kanawha Boulevard
Charleston, WV 25305
304-348-3317
*1-800-642-3671

WISCONSIN

Ms. Donna McDowell, Director
Bureau on Aging
Department of Health and
  Social Services
1 West Wilson Street, Room
  480
P.O. Box 7851
Madison, WI 53707
608-266-2536

WYOMING
Mr. Scott Sessions, Director
Commission on Aging
Hathaway Building, First
    Floor
Cheyenne, WY 82002
307-777-7986

Appendix C

Directory of Health Facility Licensing and Certification Directors

Region I: Connecticut, Maine, Massachusetts, New Hampshire, Rhode Island, Vermont

Region II: New Jersey, New York, Puerto Rico, Virgin Islands

Region III: Delaware, District of Columbia, Maryland Pennsylvania, Virginia, West Virginia

Region IV: Alabama, Florida, Georgia, Kentucky, Mississippi, North Carolina, South Carolina, Tennessee

Region V: Illinois, Indiana, Michigan, Minnesota, Ohio, Wisconsin

Region VI: Arkansas, Louisiana, New Mexico, Oklahoma, Texas

Region VII: Iowa, Kansas, Missouri, Nebraska

Region VIII: Colorado, Montana, North Dakota, South Dakota, Utah, Wyoming

Region IX: American Samoa, Arizona, California, Guam, Hawaii, Nevada

Region X: Alaska, Idaho, Oregon, Washington

REGION I
(Connecticut, Maine,
Massachusetts,
New Hampshire,
Rhode Island, Vermont)

CONNECTICUT
Elizabeth M. Burns, Director
State of Connecticut
   Department of Health
   Services
Hospital & Medical Care
   Division
150 Washington Street
Hartford, CT 06106
203-566-1073

Irene M. DiPace, Assistant
   Director
State of Connecticut
   Department of Health
   Services
Hospital & Medical Care
   Division
150 Washington Street
Hartford, CT 06106
203-566-5758

MAINE
Louis T. Dorogi, Director
Division of Licensing &
  Certification
Bureau of Medical Services
Station #11, 249 Western
  Avenue
Augusta, ME 04333
207-289-2606

MASSACHUSETTS
Patricia Plato, Director
Department of Public Health
Division of Health Care
  Quality
80 Boylston Street, Suite 1100
Boston, MA 02116
617-727-5860

Philip Dould, Assistant
  Director
Department of Public Health
Division of Health Care
  Quality
80 Boylston Street, Suite 1100
Boston, MA 02116
617-727-5860

NEW HAMPSHIRE
George P. Morse, Assistant
  Director
Division of Public Health
Office of Health Protection
6 Hazen Drive
Concord, NH 03301
603-271-4472

RHODE ISLAND
Wayne I. Farrington, Chief of
  Distribution
Rhode Island Department of
  Health
Assistant Health Program
  Administration
Facilities Regulation
75 Davis Street, Room 306
Providence, RI 02908
401-277-2566

VERMONT
Robert Aiken, Director
Medical Care Regulation
Vermont Department of
  Health
60 Main Street, Box 70
Burlington, VT 05402
802-863-7250

REGION II
(New Jersey, New York,
Puerto Rico, Virgin Islands)

NEW JERSEY
Paul R. Langevin, Jr.,
  Assistant Commissioner
New Jersey State Department
  of Health
Division of Health Facilities,
  Evaluation & Licensing
300 Whitehead Road, CN367
Trenton, NJ 08625
609-588-7732

Solomon Goldberg, D.D.S.,
  Director
Licensing, Certification,
  Standards
New Jersey State Department
  of Health
300 Whitehead Road, CN367
Trenton, NJ 08625
609-588-7726

NEW YORK
Stephen T. Berger, Director
Division of Health Care
  Standards & Surveillance
Office of Health Systems
  Management
State Department of Health
Empire State Plaza
Corning Tower, Room 1895
Albany, NY 12237
518-473-3517

Mary Jane Koran, M.D.,
   Director
Bureau of Long Term Care
   SVS
Empire State Plaza
Corning Tower, Room 1882
Albany, NY 12237
518-473-1564

PUERTO RICO
Agapito Huertas, Executive
   Director
Health & Services Facilities
   Administration
Department of Health
P.O. Box 9312
Santurce, Puerto Rico 00908

VIRGIN ISLANDS
Roy Schneider, M.D.,
   Commissioner
P.O. Box 7309
St. Thomas, Virgin Islands
   00801

REGION III
(Delaware,
District of Columbia,
Maryland, Pennsylvania,
Virginia, West Virginia)

DELAWARE
James E. Harvey, Director
Health Facilities Licensing &
   Certification
Department of Health & Social
   Services
3000 Newport Cap Pike
Wilmington, DE 19808
302-995-6674

DISTRICT OF COLUMBIA
Frances A. Bowie,
   Administrator
Dept. of Consumer &
   Regulatory Affairs
Service Facility Regulation
   Administration
614 H Street, N.W., Room
   1014
Washington, DC 20001
202-727-7190

Judith McPherson, Program
   Manager
Department of Consumer &
   Regulatory Affairs
Service Facility Regulation
   Administration
Health Facility Division
614 H Street, N.W., Room
   1014
Washington, DC 20001
202-727-7190

MARYLAND
Carol Benner, Acting Director
Office of Licensing &
   Certification Programs
Department of Health &
   Mental Hygiene
4201 Patterson Avenue
Baltimore, MD 21215-2299
301-764-2750

Gene Heisler, Deputy Director
Division of Long Term Care
Office of Licensing &
   Certification Programs
Department of Health &
   Mental Hygiene
4201 Patterson Avenue
Baltimore, MD 21215-2299
301-764-2770

PENNSYLVANIA

Andrew Major, Director
Pennsylvania Department of
  Health
Bureau of Quality Assurance
Health & Welfare Building,
  Room 907
Harrisburg, PA 17120
717-787-8015

VIRGINIA

Mary V. Francis, Director
Division of Licensure &
  Certification
Virginia Department of Health
109 Governor Street
Richmond, VA 23219
804-786-2081

WEST VIRGINIA

John J. Jarrell, Director
Department of Health and
  Human Services
Health Facility Licensure &
  Certification Section
1900 Kenawha Boulevard
  East, Building 3, Room 535
Charleston, WV 25305
304-348-0050

REGION IV

(Alabama, Florida,
Georgia, Kentucky,
Mississippi, North Carolina,
South Carolina, Tennessee)

ALABAMA

Oneal Green, Acting Director
Division of Licensure &
  Certification
Alabama Department of
  Public Health
434 Monroe Street
Montgomery, AL 36130-1701
205-261-2883

Felix F. Thornton, Deputy
  Director
Survey & Technical
  Assistance Branch
Division of Licensure &
  Certification
Alabama Department of
  Public Health
434 Monroe Street
Montgomery, AL 36130-1701
205-261-2883

FLORIDA

Connie E. Cheren, Director
Office of Licensure &
  Certification
2727 Mahan Drive
Fort Knox Building, Suite 200
Tallahassee, FL 32308
904-487-2527

GEORGIA

Dave Dunbar, Director
Standards & Licensure
Office of Regulatory Services
Georgia Department of
  Human Resources
878 Peachtree Street, N.E.,
  Room 803
Atlanta, GA 30309
404-894-5137

KENTUCKY

Woodrow Dunn, Director
Kentucky Cabinet for Human
  Resources
275 East Main Street, 4E
Frankfort, KY 40621
502-564-2800

MISSISSIPPI

Mendall G. Kemp, Director
Division of Health Facilities
Certification & Licensure
Mississippi Department of
  Health
Room 101, Underwood Annex
P.O. Box 1700
Jackson, MS 39215-1700
601-960-7769

NORTH CAROLINA
C.W. Sanders, Jr., Chief
North Carolina Department of
  Human Services
Division of Facility Services,
  Certification Secretary
701 Barbour Drive
Raleigh, NC 27603
919-733-7461

Robert I. Robeson, Chief
Medi-Med. Certification Branch
North Carolina Department of
  Human Services
Division of Facility Services
701 Barbour Drive
Raleigh, NC 27603
919-733-7461

SOUTH CAROLINA
William C. Wilkins, Director
Bureau of Certification
South Carolina Department of
  Health & Environmental
  Control
2600 Bull Street
Columbia, SC 29201
803-734-4530

Alan Samuels, Director
Office of Health Licensing
South Carolina Department of
  Health & Environmental
  Control
2600 Bull Street
Columbia, SC 29201
803-734-4680

TENNESSEE
Leslie A. Brown, Director
Health Care Facilities
Tennessee Department of
  Health & Environment
283 Plus Park Boulevard
Nashville, TN 37217
615-367-6303

H. John Bonkowski, Manager
Health Care Facilities
Tennessee Department of
  Health & Environment
283 Plus Park Boulevard
Nashville, TN 37217
615-367-6331

REGION V
(Illinois, Indiana, Michigan,
Minnesota, Ohio, Wisconsin)

ILLINOIS
Ronald L. Barth, Deputy
  Associate Director
Illinois Department of Public
  Health
525 West Jefferson, Fifth
  Floor
Springfield, IL 62761
217-782-2913
217-782-2363

Rebecca Friedman, Division
  Chief
Health Facilities Standards
Illinois Department of Public
  Health
525 West Jefferson, Fifth
  Floor
Springfield, IL 62761
217-782-7412

INDIANA
Robert Goodnow, Director
Bureau of Quality Assurance
Indiana Board of Health
1330 West Michigan Street
P.O. Box 1964
Indianapolis, IN 46206-1964
317-633-8442

Fran Pierce, Director
Division of Health Facilities
Indiana Board of Health
1330 West Michigan Street
P.O. Box 1964
Indianapolis, IN 46206-1964
317-633-8442

MICHIGAN

Evelyn K. Jones, Acting Chief
Division of Health Facility
  Licensing & Certification
Bureau of Health Facilities
Michigan Department of
  Public Health
3423 North Logan
P.O. Box 30195
Lansing, MI 48909
517-335-8506
517-335-8472

Richard D. Yerian, D.O.
Chief Medical Consultant
Bureau of Health Facilities
Michigan Department of
  Public Health
3423 North Logan
P.O. Box 30195
Lansing, MI 48909
517-335-8585
517-335-8479

MINNESOTA

H. Michael Tripple, Director
Health Resources Division
Minnesota Department of
  Health
Central Medical Building
P.O. Box 64900
393 North Dunlap Street
St. Paul, MN 55164-0900
612-643-2149

Clarice Seufert, Chief
Survey & Compliance Section
Minnesota Department of
  Health
Central Medical Building
P.O. Box 64900
393 North Dunlap Street
St. Paul, MN 55164-0900
612-643-2140

OHIO

Joseph E. Sanderell, Chief
Bureau Medical Services
Ohio Department of Health
246 North High Street
Columbus, OH 43266-0588
614-466-7857

Howard "Don" Donahue,
  Assistant Chief
Bureau Medical Services
Ohio Department of Health
246 North High Street
Columbus, OH 43266-0588
614-466-2070

WISCONSIN

Larry Tainter, Director
Bureau of Quality Compliance
Wisconsin Division of Health
P.O. Box 309
Madison, WI 53701
608-267-7185

Susan Wood, Deputy Director
Bureau of Quality Compliance
Wisconsin Division of Health
P.O. Box 309
Madison, WI 53701
608-266-8472

REGION VI
(Arkansas, Louisiana,
New Mexico, Oklahoma,
Texas)

ARKANSAS

Bobbie M. Brown, R.N.
Arkansas Department of
  Health
4815 W. Markham Street
Little Rock, AR 72205-3867
501-661-2201

Valetta M. Buck, Director
Division of Health Facilities
   Services
Arkansas Department of
   Health
4815 West Markham Street
Little Rock, AR 72205-3867
501-661-2201

LOUISIANA

Steve Phillips, Director
Division of Licensing &
   Certification
Department of Health &
   Hospitals
P.O. Box 3767
Baton Rouge, LA 70821
504-342-5774

George T. Jones, Assistant
   Director
Division of Licensing &
   Certification
Department of Health &
   Hospitals
P.O. Box 3767
Baton Rouge, LA 70821
504-342-5774

NEW MEXICO

Sue K. Morris, Bureau Chief
Health Facility Licensing &
   Certification Bureau
Health Services Division
New Mexico Health
   Environment Department
1190 St. Francis Drive
Harold Runnels Building, N-
   1400
Santa Fe, NM 87503
505-827-2409
505-827-2413

Matthew Gervase, Supervisor
Federal Program Certification
   Section
New Mexico Health
   Environment Department
1190 St. Francis Drive
Harold Runnels Building, N-
   1350
Santa Fe, NM 87503
505-827-2416
505-827-2427

OKLAHOMA

Brent E. VanMeter, Deputy
   Commissioner of Health
Special Health Services
Oklahoma State Department
   of Health
1000 N.E. Tenth
P.O. Box 53551
Oklahoma City, OK 73152
405-271-4200

Evelyn Battle, Chief
Special Health Services, Long-
   Term Care Division
Oklahoma State Department
   of Health
1000 N.E. Tenth
P.O. Box 53551
Oklahoma City, OK 73152
405-271-6868

TEXAS

Juanita Carrell, Associate
   Commissioner
Special Health Services
Texas Department of Health
1100 West 49th Street
Austin, TX 78756-3197
512-458-7296

Jerry W. Bryant, Director
Quality Standards Division
Texas Department of Health
1100 West 49th Street
Austin, TX 78756-3197
512-458-7611

REGION VII
(Iowa, Kansas, Missouri,
Nebraska)

IOWA
Dana L. Petrowsky,
Administrator
Division of Health Facilities
Iowa Department of Inspection
& Appeals
Health Facilities Division
Lucas State Office Building
Des Moines, IA 50319
515-281-4115
515-281-4294

Mary Oliver, Executive
Assistant
Division of Health Facilities
Iowa Department of Inspection
& Appeals
Health Facilities Division
Lucas State Office Building
Des Moines, IA 50319
515-281-4115
515-281-4081

KANSAS
Richard J. Morrissey, Bureau
Director of Adult & Child
Care
Kansas Department of Health
& Environment
900 S.W. Jackson, Suite
#1001
Landon Street Office Building
Topeka, KS 66612-1290
913-296-1240

MISSOURI
J. Barton Boyle, Director
Bureau of Hospital Licensing
& Certification
Missouri Department of Health
1738 East Elm Street
P.O. Box 570
Jefferson City, MO 65102
314-751-6302

Lois Kollmeyer, R.N., Chief
Bureau of Home Health
Licensing & Certification
Missouri Department of Health
1738 East Elm Street
P.O. Box 570
Jefferson City, MO 65102
314-751-6336

NEBRASKA
William H. Page, Director
Department of Health
Division of Licensure &
Standards
301 Centennial Mall South
Lincoln, NB 68509
402-471-2946

REGION VIII
(Colorado, Montana,
North Dakota, South Dakota,
Utah, Wyoming)

COLORADO
Mildred G. Simmons, Director
Health Facilities Division
Colorado Department of
Health
4210 East Eleventh Avenue
Denver, CO 80220
303-331-4990
303-393-4928

Diane Carter, Director
Support & Analysis
Health Facilities Division
Colorado Department of
Health
4210 East Eleventh Avenue
Denver, CO 80220
303-331-4990
303-331-4971

MONTANA

J. Dale Taliaferro,
    Administrator
Health Sciences Division
Montana Department of
    Health & Environment
Cogswell Building, Room
    C214
Helena, MT 59620
406-444-4473

Denzel C. Davis
Licensing & Certification
    Bureau
Montana Department of
    Health & Environment
Cogswell Building, Room
    C214
Helena, MT 59620
406-444-2037

NORTH DAKOTA

Fred Gladden, Chief
Health Resources Section
North Dakota State
    Department of Health
State Capitol Judicial Wing,
    Second Floor
600 East Boulevard Avenue
Bismark, ND 58505-0200
701-224-2352

Dorrene Haugrud, Survey
    Process Manager
Division of Health Facilities
North Dakota State
    Department of Health
State Capitol Judicial Wing,
    Second Floor
600 East Boulevard Avenue
Bismark, ND 58505-0200
701-224-2352

SOUTH DAKOTA

Sue Lydic, Program Director
Licensure & Certification
    Program
523 East Capitol, Joe Foss
    Building
Pierre, SD 57501
605-773-3364

Mike Baker, Deputy Director
Licensure & Certification
    Program
523 East Capitol, Joe Foss
    Building
Pierre, SD 57501
605-773-3364

UTAH

Allan D. Elkins, Director
Bureau of Facility Review
Utah Department of Health
288 North 1460 West
Salt Lake City, UT 84116-
    0660
801-538-6559
801-538-6595

James B. Fisher, Director
Bureau of Facilities Licensure
Utah Department of Health
288 North 1460 West
Salt Lake City, UT 84116-
    0660
801-538-6152
801-538-6320

WYOMING

Charles Simineo, Program
    Manager
Division of Health & Medical
    Services
Hathaway Building, Fourth
    Floor
Cheyenne, WY 82002
307-777-7121

REGION IX
(American Samoa, Arizona, California, Guam, Hawaii, Nevada)

AMERICAN SAMOA
Julia L. Lyons, M.D., MPH
Director of Health
Health Services Regulatory
  Board
Pago Pago, AS 96799
684-633-1222

(No licensure and certification activities in this territory.)

ARIZONA
Berry Singleton, M.D.
Health Care Licensure
701 East Jefferson, Suite 300
Phoenix, AZ 85034
602-255-1177

Wilburt Nelson, Acting
  Program Manager
Health Care Licensure
701 East Jefferson, Suite 300
Phoenix, AZ 85034
602-255-1177

CALIFORNIA
Teresa Hawkes, Deputy
  Director
Department of Health Services
Licensing & Certification
  Division
714 "P" Street, Room 823
Sacramento, CA 95814
916-445-3054
916-445-2070

Paul H. Keller, Chief
Department of Health Services
714 "P" Street, Room 823
Sacramento, CA 95814
916-445-2070
916-324-8625

GUAM
Vincente D. Quitoriano, R.S.
  Administrator
Department of Public Health
  & Social Services
P.O. Box 2816
Agana, Guam 96910
671-734-2671

Logan C. Oplinger,
  Environmental Health
  Specialist
Department of Public Health
  & Social Services
Agana, Guam 96910
671-734-3671

HAWAII
Benjamin Lambiotte, M.D.,
  Chief
Hospital & Medical Facilities
  Branch
Department of Health
P.O. Box 3378
Honolulu, HI 96801
808-548-5935

Elizabeth K. Anderson, M.D.,
  Chief
Medical Health Services
  Division
Department of Health
P.O. Box 3378
Honolulu, HI 96801
808-548-6510

NEVADA
William C. Schneider, Bureau
  Chief
Bureau of Regulatory Health
  Services
505 East King Street, Room
  202
Carson City, NV 89710
702-885-4475

George E. Reynolds, M.D.
Medical Director
505 East King Street, Room
    202
Carson City, NV 89710
702-885-4475

REGION X
(Alaska, Idaho, Oregon,
Washington)

ALASKA
Karen Martz, Administrator
Office of Health Facilities
    Licensing & Certification
Department of Health & Social
    Services
4433 Business Park Boulevard
Anchorage, AK 99503-0333
907-561-2171

IDAHO
Jean Schoonover, R.N., Chief
Bureau of Facility Standards
Department of Health &
    Welfare
450 West State Street, Second
    Floor
Boise, ID 83720-9990
208-334-6626

Loyal I. Perry, Supervisor
Licensing & Certification
Bureau of Facility Standards,
    Health & Welfare
450 West State Street, Second
    Floor
Boise, ID 83720-9990
208-334-6627

OREGON
Jill Laney, Manager
Health Facilities Section
Health Division
1400 S.W. Fifth Avenue,
    Room 605
Portland, OR 97201
503-229-5348

D.J. Kramer, Manager
Client Care Monitoring Unit
Senior Services Division
313 Public Services Building
Salem, OR 97310
503-373-7163

WASHINGTON
Ken Lewis, Manager
Health Facilities Survey
    Section
MS ET-321
1112 South Quince
Olympia, WA 98504
206-753-5851

Cathy Wiggins, Director
Nursing Home Services,
    DSHS, AASA
623 Eighth Avenue S.E.
Mail Stop HB-11
Olympia, WA 98504-0095
206-753-4465

Appendix D

Resource Centers for the Needs and Concerns of the Elderly

ACTION
100 Vermont Avenue, NW,
  6th Floor
Washington, DC 20525
(federal agency administering
  senior volunteer programs)

ADRDA (Alzheimer's Disease
  and Related Disorders
  Association, Inc.)
70 East Lake Street, Suite
  600
Chicago, IL 60601
(brochures and general information)

AARP (American Association
  of Retired Persons)
1909 K Street
Washington, DC 20049
(general information and locations of activity programs)

Administration on Aging
330 Independence Avenue,
  SW
Washington, DC 20201
(interested in complaints and
  quality of care in nursing
  homes)

Aids Clearing House
P.O. Box 6003
Rockville, MD 20850 (1-800-
  458-5231)
(general information, referrals,
  and resources)

American Association of
  Homes for the Aging
1129 20th Street, NW, Suite
  400
Washington, DC 20036
(membership organization for
  non-proprietary homes; general information and publications)

American Health Care
  Association
1201 L Street, NW
Washington, DC 20005-4014
(membership organization of
  proprietary homes; general
  information; publishes special reports and surveys)

American Cancer Society-
National Office
1599 Clifton Road, NE
Atlanta, GA 30329
(general literature, information,
and addresses of local chapters)

American College of Health
Care Administrators
325 South Patrick Street
Alexandria, VA 22314
(interested in complaints regarding nursing home ad-
ministrators)

American Foundation for the
Blind
15 West 16th Street
New York, NY 10011
(general information and brochures)

American Parkinson's Disease
Association, Inc.
116 John Street
New York, NY 10034
(general information, brochures, and literature)

American Psychological
Association
1200 17th Street, NW
Washington, DC 20036
(counseling, referrals, and resources)

County Medical Societies
(listed in local phone books and
libraries; provides names of
physicians; also interested in
complaints regarding spe-
cific doctors)

County Offices of Consumer
Affairs
(listed in local phone books and
libraries; interested in complaints about specific nursing homes; provides general
information on local facilities)

Department of Health and
Human Services
Health Care and Financing
Administration
6325 Security Boulevard
Baltimore, MD 21207
(federal guidelines and standards governing nursing centers)

Department of Health and
Human Services
Social Security Administration
6401 Security Boulevard
Baltimore, MD 21235
(general information on Medicare)

Gerontological Society
1275 K Street, NW
Washington, DC 20005
(general information on the elderly)

Grey Panthers National Office
311 Juniper Street
Philadelphia, PA 19107
(general information and brochures)

JCAH (Joint Commission on
Accreditation of Hospitals)
875 North Michigan Avenue
Chicago, IL 60611
(interested in complaints about
member nursing centers)

Institute of Medicine
2101 Constitution Avenue, NW
Washington, DC 20418
(Nursing Home Study Commission issues recommendations on national health policy; provides publications.)

National Association of Boards of Examiners for Nursing Home Administrators
808 17th Street, NW, Suite 200
Washington, DC 20006
(issues names, addresses, and phone numbers of each state's regulatory agency for nursing home administrators)

National Citizens' Coalition for Nursing Home Reform
1424 16th Street, Suite L2
Washington, DC 20036
(citizens' group involvement in nursing home issues)

National Consumer League
815 15th Street, NW, Suite 516
Washington, DC 20005
(interested in the quality of care in nursing homes)

National Council on the Aging
600 Maryland Avenue SW, West Wing 100
Washington, DC 20024
(interested in complaints about specific nursing homes)

The following Institutes come under the heading of the National Institutes of Health (NIH). The goal of NIH is the improvement of the health of the American people by supporting medical research, research training, and the development of research resources.

National Institute on Aging
9000 Rockville Pike
Bethesda, MD 20892
(conducts biomedical and behavioral research to increase knowledge about aging; memory loss, incontinence, and susceptibility to diseases are areas of special concern)

National Institute of Allergy and Infectious Diseases
9000 Rockville Pike
Bethesda, MD 20892
(general information on asthma, immunology, venereal diseases, organ transplants, hepatitis, influenza, and other viral respiratory infections)

National Institute of Neurological and Communicative Disorders and Stroke
9000 Rockville Pike
Bethesda, MD 20892
(general information; conducts research on Parkinson's disease, epilepsy, multiple sclerosis, head and spinal cord injuries, disorders of speech, deafness, and stroke)

National Eye Institute
9000 Rockville Pike
Bethesda, MD 20892
(general information on eye and visual system diseases)

Additional information, addresses and phone numbers on the National Institutes and other United States Government Agencies can be obtained by writing:

> Office of the Federal Register
> National Archives and Records Administration
> Washington, DC 20408

The Federal Register is issued each federal working day and provides information on the presidential and regulatory documents. (Contact the reference section of the local library.)

The Code of Federal Regulations is an annual codification of the rules published in the Federal Register. It is divided into fifty titles and is kept up to date by the issues of the Federal Register. (Contact the reference section of the local library.)

Publications of the Office of the Federal Register are available for sale by writing:

> Superintendent of Documents
> Government Printing Office,
> Washington, DC 20402.

Documents especially pertaining to aging can be obtained by writing:

> Documents
> Special Committee on Aging
> SD-G31, Dirksen Building U.S. Senate
> Washington, DC 20510

To obtain information on recent bills regarding nursing home issues, write to:

> United States House of Representatives
> Washington, DC 20515
>   and
> United States Senate
> Washington, DC 20510

United States Congressional Offices (general information number): (202) 224-3121

Appendix E

Drugs in Geriatrics

Many different medications are used in geriatrics. However, certain medications are more commonly ordered by physicians than others. The ones most commonly used, their effects, and generic names are listed on pages 165-166. However, before you look up any specific medication and its use, it is important to know that there are different ways of giving medicines. For instance, a medication might be given by mouth in pill form but, if the patient cannot take the medicine in pill form, it might be given in an easier-to-swallow form, as a liquid. Injections or suppositories might also be used when other methods fail or cannot be tolerated. For instance, it is sometimes necessary to give anti-nausea medications by suppository or injection when a resident has nausea due to the flu.

Years ago, when medications were not available in forms other than the tablet, it was common practice for nurses to crush medications and give them in applesauce, ice cream, jelly, or at mealtimes in food. Not only did crushing the pills destroy the protective coverings designed to prevent irritation in the stomach, but many residents developed an aversion to their food when medicines were given in this way. Over the years new administration methods have made this technique not only unnecessary but also frowned upon by health professionals.

Not every medication can be given in the same form. Some drugs can be given by mouth, in pill or in liquid form, and others, such as nitroglycerine and certain hormones, can be used topically. Anti-motion-sickness drugs can be applied to a patch which is worn behind the ear. Some medications can also be used as ointments, creams, and lotions, and still others can be given by aerosol.

Continual research on new and better ways to administer drugs is being conducted, and in the future it is possible that certain medications will be administered by way of eye or nose drops.

The following medications, the ones most commonly used in geriatrics, are listed by trade name, followed by their effects, and their generic names.

Medications Most Commonly Used in Geriatrics

Trade Name	Effects	Generic Name
Adapin	antidepressant	doxepin
Aldactone	diuretic	spironolactone
Aldactazide	diuretic	spironolactone/HCTZ
Aldomet	reduces blood pressure	methyldopa
Antivert	lessens dizziness and motion sickness	meclizine
Apresoline	decreases blood pressure	hydralazine
Ascriptin	relieves pain	aspirin
Ativan	decreases anxiety	lorazepam
AVC cream	treats vaginal infections	sulfanilamide, aminacrine HCL
Aventyl	antidepressant	nortriptyline
Benadryl	antihistamine; sleep aid	diphenhydramine
Betadine Ung.	antisepsis	povidone-iodine
Brethine/ Bricanyl	bronchodilator	terbutaline sulfate
Chronulac	laxative	lactulose
Cogentin	anti-Parkinson drug	benztropine mesylate
Colbenemid	treats gouty arthritis	colchicine/probenecid
Compazine	tranquilizer/anti-nausea and vomiting	prochlorperazine
Coumadin	anti-clotting agent	warfarin
Darvon	analgesic	propoxyphene HCL
Darvon Compound	analgesic	propoxyphene with aspirin and caffeine
Desyrel	antidepressant	trazodone
Dilantin	anti-seizures	phenytoin
Diuril	decreases blood pressure; diuretic	chlorthiazide
Dopar	anti-Parkinson's disease	levodopa
Dulcolax	laxative	bisacodyl
Dyazide	decreases blood pressure; diuretic	hydrochlorothiazide/ triamterene
Elavil	antidepressant	amitriptyline
Eskolith lithane	treats manic depression	lithium carbonate
Feosol	increases iron in blood	ferrous sulfate
Gantrisin	treats infections	sulfisoxozole
Glucatrol	antidiabetic	glipizide
Halcion	sleep aid	triazolam
Haldol	tranquilizer	haloperidol

Medications Most Commonly Used in Geriatrics

Trade Name	Effects	Generic Name
Hydergine	mood elevator used in Alzheimer's disease	ergoloid mesylates
Hydrodiuril	diuretic; decreases blood pressure	hydrochorthiazide
Hygroton	diuretic; decreases blood pressure	chlorthalidone
Inderal	decreases blood pressure	propranolol
Kaon/Klorvess K-Lor	increases potassium	potassium chloride
Lanoxin	treats heart arrhythmias	digoxin
Lasix	diuretic/decreases blood pressure	furosemide
Lidex cream	treats dermatitis	fluocinonide
Lomotil	anti-diarrheal	diphenoxylate
Mellaril	tranquilizer	thioridazine HCL
Metamucil	laxative	psyllium
MOM	laxative	magnesium
Motrin	anti-inflammatory	ibuprofen
Nitro-Dur patch	anti-angina	nitroglycerine
Nitro-Bid	anti-angina	nitroglycerine
Orinase	antidiabetic	tolbutamide
Peri-Colace	laxative	docusate sodium casanthranol
Prozac	antidepressant	fluoxetine
Quinaglute	anti-arrhythmic (heart)	quinidine gluconate
Ritalin	antidepressant, stimulant	methylphenidate
Septra/ Bactrim	anti-infective	sulfamethoxazole/ trimethoprim
Sinemet	anti-Parkinson	levodopa
Sinequan	antidepressant	doxepin HCL
Slo-Phyllin	bronchodilator	theophylline
Synthroid	thyroid replacement	levothyroxine
Tagamet	treats ulcers	cimetidine
Theodur	bronchodilator	theophylline
Thorazine	tranquilizer	chlorpromazine
Tofranil	anti-depressive	imipramine
Tolinase	anti-diabetic	tolazamide
Tylenol	analgesic	acetaminophen
Zantac	treats ulcers	ranitidine
Zyloprim	treats gouty arthritis	allopurinol

The group of drugs called *antacids* are so widely used and of such variety that I have chosen to handle these separately and list them by their ingredients. These medications are used to neutralize excess acid in the stomach. Some of these medications can cause symptoms such as constipation and/or diarrhea, depending on the ingredients.

Antacids containing calcium, which can cause constipation: Calcium Carbonate and Tums.

Antacids containing aluminum, which might cause constipation: Rolaids and Alternagel.

Symptoms of diarrhea can occur with the following: Milk of Magnesia, Aludrox, Maalox, Riopan, Camalox, Digel, Gelusil, Maalox Plus, and Mylanta.

All antacids should be given one to two hours before or after other drugs, as they may interfere with the absorption of such other medications as Dilantin, Digoxin, and Quinidine.

The narcotic analgesics most often used in nursing homes are: Demerol, Morphine, Percodan, Numorphan, Percocet, and Tylenol #3.

There are many new preparations on the market that are used in nursing homes, but the above drugs are among those that are most frequently used.

Glossary of Medical Terms

Abrasion: Scraped skin.

Abuse: Mistreatment of a resident in a nursing home. Can be physical, verbal, and/or emotional.

Acquired Immune Deficiency Syndrome (AIDS): Disease caused by a virus which progressively disrupts the body's immune system.

Activities of Daily Living (ADLS): Dressing, bathing, mobility, continence, and feeding.

Acute: Sudden attack of a disease or stage of a disease.

Adjudicate: Final determination by a judge or other competent authority. Example: adjudication of a resident as mentally incompetent.

Affect: Emotional feeling and mood.

AIDS Related Complex (ARC): Symptoms include fever, swollen glands, weight loss, and infections. Not all patients with this disease develop AIDS.

Alzheimer's disease: Most common cause of dementia, characterized by symptoms of loss of memory, confusion, and disorientation.

Ambulation: Walking.

Analgesic: Any method used to relieve pain, such as oral and/or injectable medications, ointments, or compresses.

Aneurysm: Dilation of an artery due to weakness of the tissue or pressure from blood on the walls of the vessel.

Angina pectoris: Chest pain. Commonly felt as a squeezing or pressing discomfort.

Anorexia: Decreased appetite.

Antiseptic: Substance that prevents or stops the growth of infectious material. Example: alcohol or povidone.

Arteriosclerosis: Hardening of the walls of the arteries.

Ascites: Fluid in the abdomen due to kidney, heart, or liver disease.

Aseptic: Germfree.

Ataxia: Uncoordinated walking.

Bedsore (pressure sore): Pressure area on a part of body. Classified in stages I–IV: Stage I—redness; Stage II—redness and an open area; Stage III—open area down to subcutaneous layer; Stage IV—open area, with necrosis and/or eschar; can involve bone.

Benign: Not malignant.

Bradycardia: Very slow heart beat.

Bronchi: Divisions of the trachea.

Bronchial: Refers to the bronchi.

Bronchitis: Inflammation of the bronchi.

Bronchospasm: Spasms of the bronchi.

Bowel and bladder training program: Retraining bowel and bladder functions. A resident is taken to the bathroom on a regular schedule to help regulate elimination.

Butterfly: Small adhesive covering used to close a wound; sometimes used instead of sutures.

Cachexia: Wasting away.

Calculi: Stones, such as kidney or gallbladder stones.

Catheter: A tube inserted into an opening in the body, such as the bladder, rectum, or stomach, to evacuate or inject fluids. Most often refers to a tube used to drain urine from the bladder.

Carcinoma: Malignancy.

Cerebrovascular accident (CVA): Stroke.

Certified medicine aide (CMA): One who completes a training course, passes an exam, and is certified to dispense medications.

Chemical restraints: Medications used as a means of controlling a behavior, such as agitation—as opposed to medications used to treat the cause of the agitation.

Chronic: Long-standing (ongoing) disease or condition, such as chronic bronchitis.

Chronic obstructive pulmonary disease (COPD): Irreversible obstruction of airways. The most common obstructive pulmonary disease in nursing centers is emphysema.

Colitis: Inflammation of the colon that usually results in loose bowel movements and causes cramps, nausea and/or vomiting, and sometimes blood in the bowel movement.

Colostomy: Artificial anus made on the outside of the abdomen that allows elimination of the bowels.

Complete blood count (CBC): Blood test in which cells and other blood substances are counted. Should be done routinely on residents who are on medication that may cause a disturbance of the blood cells or to detect anemia, other diseases, and/or infection.

Congestive heart failure (CHF): Refers to the heart failing in its output, resulting in pulmonary congestion or fluid collection in other parts of the body.

Continent: Voluntary control of output of feces and/or urine.

Contracture: Rigid, stiff joint; results in loss of movement in this area.

Debridement: Excision of dead tissue from a bedsore or wound.

Decubitus (pressure sore): Bedsore. (See stages of, under definition of bedsore.)

Dementia: General deterioration of mental function due to organic or psychological factors.

Dermatitis: Rash, sometimes with itching.

Disorientation: Confusion as to time, place, and person.

Diuretic: Anything that causes increased urination.

Dressing: Protective covering, or bandage.

Dyskinesia: Involuntary extraneous movements. Can be a side effect of a drug or may be a symptom of a disease.

Edema: Accumulation of fluid in body tissues, especially in extremities.

Egg crate: Foam mattress or chair pad with areas of peaks and valleys resembling an egg carton.

Emesis: Vomiting.

Emphysema: A chronic pulmonary disease resulting in enlargement of air spaces and destructive changes in the tissues, most frequently caused by cigarette smoking.

Erythema: Redness of the skin.

Eschar: Necrotic (dead) tissue.

Etiology: Cause of a disease.

Febrile: Condition of elevated body temperature.

Femur: Thigh bone.

Federal standard: Refers to a federal rule and/or regulation.

Gait: Refers to walking.

Gangrene: Dead skin and tissue.

Gastric: Refers to the stomach.

Gastrostomy: An opening into the stomach. When a tube is inserted directly into the stomach through an incision in the skin, it is called a "G tube."

Generic drugs: Medicines having the same chemical ingredients as their equivalent brand-name drugs but usually priced lower. Usually, but not necessarily, therapeutically equivalent.

Geriatric nurse assistant: Nursing assistant employed in a nursing home.

Gout: Metabolic condition in which uric acid builds up to abnormally high levels. Uric acid deposits may result in "gouty arthritis."

Heel pads: Protective coverings used on the heels of a resident to prevent friction and skin breakdown. Can be made of foam, lambswool, or any material that acts as a cushion.

Hematuria: Blood in the urine. May be microscopic (seen only by laboratory examination) or gross (visibly bloody).

H_2O mattress: A special mattress filled with water and used as a protection against skin breakdown.

Hepatic: Refers to the liver.

Herpes simplex: Cold sore caused by a specific virus.

Herpes zoster: Shingles; caused by the same virus that causes chicken pox.

Hour of Sleep (HS): Bedtime.

Hypoxia: Decreased oxygen in the blood.

Immune: Resistant to a disease.

Immune system: Body's defense system.

Incontinence: Lack of voluntary control of either bowel or bladder.

Incontinence pads: Disposable or other material used to absorb bladder or bowel matter.

Intermediate care facility (ICF): Nursing home that provides a level of care that is less than skilled but provides more than simply room and board.

IV: Abbreviation for "intravenous."

Kaposi's sarcoma: Reddish, purple tumor, associated with AIDS. Usually begins on the lower extremities and spreads to other parts of the body.

Kyphosis: Curved spine, giving the appearance of a humpback.

Laceration: Skin tear.

Lethargy: Drowsiness.

Level of care: Refers to the specific kind of medical care a resident receives, such as skilled, intermediate, or chronic.

Licensed practical nurse (LPN): One who has taken a required course and passed an examination.

Lipoma: Benign fatty tumor.

Lithiasis: Calculi (stones), such as kidney stones, known as nephrolithiasis, or gallstones (cholelithiasis).

Malignant: Cancerous, as opposed to benign.

Manic depression: A mental disease characterized by alternating periods of agitation and depression.

Medicaid: The state federal program that pays for the medical care of the indigent and is authorized by Title XIX of the Social Security Act.

Medicare: The federally funded program for those sixty-five years old and over, or permanently and totally disabled, and authorized by Title XVIII of the Social Security Act. Consists of Parts A and B.

Medicare Part A: Refers to hospital and skilled nursing home benefits. Financed by Social Security trust funds; has a deductible and a co-payment.

Medicare Part B: Refers to physicians' services, outpatient therapies, some medical supplies, and home health benefits. An optional plan that has a monthly premium and a deductible.

Metastasis: The spread of a disease such as cancer from one site to another.

Nasogastric feeding (NG): Refers to the feeding that is given through a tube inserted into the stomach through the nose.

O$_2$: Oxygen.

Ombudsman: Advocate, authorized under Title III of the Older Americans Act, who investigates residents' complaints, monitors rules and regulations in nursing homes, and provides information to public agencies regarding residents' problems.

Orthopedic: Refers to the bones.

Osteomyelitis: Infection of a bone.

Otic: Refers to the ear.

OTC: Abbreviation for "over the counter."

Parallel bars: Physical therapy device used to retrain a resident in walking.

Parkinson's disease: Progressive disease of a portion of the brain. Some symptoms include muscle stiffness, slow body movement, and tremors of extremities. Major tranquilizers may cause similar symptoms.

Pathological fracture: Break in a bone which occurs because the bone is diseased.

Patient care plan: Program of care instituted by nurse and physician, and added to by a multidisciplinary team. The plan lists problems and approaches to attain specific goals in the resident's care.

Pedal edema: Swelling of feet and ankles usually from accumulation of fluid.

Per os (P.O.): By mouth. Example: a doctor's order may read "give medication per os."

Personal physician: Resident's primary, or attending, doctor.

Podiatry: Foot care.

PRN: Abbreviation which may follow an order for a medication used "only when needed." Example: a doctor's order may read "Aspirin, 5 grains, every 4 hrs., prn for pain."

Protective device: Items such as belts, vests, or mittens used to protect a resident from self-injury or injury to someone else.

Pulmonary: Refers to the lungs.

Rales: Abnormal bubbling sound heard in the lungs.

Range of motion (ROM): The degree to which a limb can be moved. Also, therapy designed to improve a limb's function.

Reality orientation: Communication approach used to familiarize a confused resident with surroundings, time, and identity.

Registered nurse (RN): One who is licensed by the state after completing an educational program of at least two years and passing an examination.

Rehabilitative: Therapeutic measures, such as range-of-motion, physical, speech, occupational, and recreational therapies, used to restore lost function.

Restorative measures: Therapeutic techniques or methods, such as range-of-motion therapy, used to regain function.

Sarcoma: Malignant tumor of muscle.

Senescence: Aging.

Senile dementia: Formerly used as a synonym for Alzheimer's disease.

Sheepskin: Padding used between a resident's body and a hard item such as a chair, for protection against skin injury.

Skilled nursing facility (SNF): Nursing home that provides a level of care less than an acute hospital but more than an intermediate nursing home.

Staph infection: Infection due to the staphylococcus organism; a frequent cause of boils, abscesses, and purulent wound infections.

Stat: Immediately.

Sub-lingual (SL): A method of administering medication under the tongue.

Supplementary Medical Insurance Program—Part B: Medicare Part B; covers physicians' services, outpatient therapy, some medical supplies, and home health visits.

Suppository: Medication administered rectally or vaginally.

Suprapubic cystotomy: Surgical opening of the bladder to the skin above the pubic bone. A catheter inserted into this opening is known as a "suprapubic cystostomy."

Tachycardia: Rapid heart beat.

TPR: Abbreviation for temperature, pulse, and respirations.

Therapeutic: Possesses healing potential.

Thrombus: Blood clot.

Tracheotomy: Opening into the trachea. A tube inserted into this opening is known as a tracheostomy.

Transient-ischemic attack (TIA): Resembles a stroke and is often called a "mini-stroke."

Unguent (ung.): Salve.

Uric Acid: Chemical crystals.

Urology: Study of diseases related to the urinary system.

UTI: Abbreviation for "urinary tract infection."

Vaginitis: Inflammation of vagina.

Vertigo: Dizziness.

Virus: Microscopic organisms which can infect the body.

Bibliography

A Brief Explanation of Medicare. Social Security Administration. SSA Publication No. 05-10043.

Beletz, Elaine E., R.N., and Gabriel A. Covo, M.D. "The Case of the Hidden Infections in the Elderly." *Nursing 76.* August 1976, pp. 15–16.

Berkow, Robert, M.D., ed. *Merck Manual of Diagnosis and Therapy.* 15th ed. Rahway, N.J.: Merck Sharp & Dohme Research Laboratories, 1987.

Billig, Nathan, M.D. *To Be Old and Sad: Understanding Depression in the Elderly.* Lexington, Mass.: Lexington Books, 1987.

Bowlby, John. *Attachment and Loss.* Vol. 3: *Loss, Sadness, and Depression.* New York: Basic Books, Harper and Row, 1980.

Carlson, Eugene. "New Study Looks at the State of Nation's 'Old-Old' Citizens." *Wall Street Journal.* 5 August 1986, p. 33.

Code of Federal Regulations. Title 42. Chapter IV. Part 405. 1985.

Code of Federal Regulations. Title 42. Chapter IV. Parts 442.1–442.346. 1985.

Cohen, Donna, Ph.D., and Carl Eisdorfer, Ph.D., M.D. *The Loss of Self.* New York: W. W. Norton, 1986.

Cohn, Victor. "Making Sure Your Last Wishes Are Followed." *Washington Post*, Health Section. 1 March 1988, p. 14.

Colburn, Don. "Facing the Certainty of Death." *Washington Post*, Health Section. 14 April 1987, p. 18.

Colburn, Don. "Numbers in Nursing Homes Expected to Soar by 2025." *Washington Post*, Health Section. 27 June 1989, p. 5.

Consumers Guide to Medicare Supplement Insurance. Health Insurance Association. Write to: 1025 Connecticut Avenue, Washington, D.C. 20036. June 1989.

Cornacchia, Harold J., Ed.D., and Stephen Barrett, M.D. *Shopping for Health Care: The Essential Guide to Products and Services.* New York: Mosby Press, 1982.

Coville, Walter J., Timothy W. Costello, and Fabian L. Rouka. *Abnormal Psychology.* New York: Barnes and Noble, 1960.

Dunlop, Burton, ed. *Growth of Nursing Home Care.* Lexington, Mass.: Heath Publishers, 1979.

Feil, Naomi. "Communicating with the Confused Elderly Patient." *Geriatrics.* Vol. 39, no. 3. March 1984, p. 131.

Freedman, Alex M. "Nursing Homes Try New Approach in Caring for Alzheimer's Victims." *Wall Street Journal.* 26 September 1986.

Freese, Arthur S. *Stroke: The New Hope and the New Help.* New York: Random House, 1980.

Gwyther, Lisa P. *Care of Alzheimer's Patients: A Manual for Nursing Home Staff.* Washington, D.C.: American Health Care Association and the Alzheimer's Disease and Related Disorders Association, 1985.

The Health Education Resource Organization. *AIDS and the Nursing Home Patient.* Washington, D.C.: The American Health Care Association and The National Foundation for Long-Term Health Care, October 1985.

Heifetz, Milton D., and Charles Mangel. *The Right to Die.* New York: G.P. Putnam's Sons, 1985.

Hendler, Nelson H., M.D., and Judith Fenton. *Coping with Chronic Pain.* New York: Clarkson N. Potter, 1979.

Institute of Medicine Committee on Nursing Home Regulation. *Improving the Quality of Care in Nursing Homes.* Washington, D.C.: National Academy Press, 1986.

Islatt, James I., M.D., and John K. Brubaker. *The AIDS Epidemic.* New York: Warner Books, 1985.

Johnson, Colleen L., and Leslie A. Grant. *The Nursing Home in American Society.* Baltimore: Johns Hopkins University Press, 1985.

Kastrup, Erwin K., B.S. Pharmacy, ed. *Facts and Comparisons.* St . Louis, Missouri: Gene H. Schwach for J.B. Lippincott, 1988.

Keenan, Maryanne P. "Changing Needs for Long-Term Care: A Chart Book." Washington, D.C.: Public Policy Institute, American Association of Retired Persons, 1989.

Knowing Your Rights: Medicare's Prospective Payment System. American Association of Retired Persons. Write to: Fulfillment, 1909 K Street, Washington, D.C. 20049.

Kübler-Ross, Elizabeth, M.D. *On Death and Dying.* New York: MacMillan, 1969.

Kushner, Irving, M.D. *Understanding Arthritis.* New York: Charles Scribner's Sons, 1984.

Lewin, Tamar. "Nursing Homes Rethink Merits of Tying the Aged." *New York Times,* Section B. 28 December, 1989, p. 1.

Lieberman, M. Laurence. *The Essential Guide to Generic Drugs.* New York: Harper and Row, 1986.

Mace, Nancy L., and Peter V. Rabins. *The 36-Hour Day.* Baltimore: Johns Hopkins University Press, 1981.

McDonald, Thomas F., *Target: Tomorrow: Quality of Life for Residential Elders*. Washington, D.C.: American Health Care Association, 1982.

Morris, William, ed. *American Heritage Dictionary of the English Language*. New York: American Heritage and Houghton Mifflin, 1969.

National Citizens' Coalition for Nursing Home Reform. "Illinois Supreme Court Upholds 1979 Nursing Home Reform Act." *Quality Care Advocate*. July/August 1986.

National Citizens' Coalition for Nursing Home Reform. "Congress Passes Quality Care Bill; Major Reforms Become Law at Last." *Quality Care Advocate*. January/February 1988.

On the Other Side of Easy Street: Myths and Facts about the Economics of Old Age. Write to: The Villars Foundation, 1334 G Street, N.W. Washington, D.C. 20005.

Pear, Robert. "New Law Protects Rights of Patients in Nursing Homes." *New York Times*, Section 1. 17 January 1988, p. 1.

Perish, Peter, M.D. *The Doctor's and Patient's Handbook of Medicines and Drugs*. 2nd ed., rev. New York: Alfred A. Knopf, 1980.

Powell, Lenora S., and Katie Courtic. *Alzheimer's Disease: A Guide for Families*. Reading, Mass.: Addison-Wesley, 1983.

Pritchard, Vicki, R.N., M.S.N., C.I.C. "Preventing and Treating Geriatric Infections." *RN*. March 1988, pp. 36–38.

Rich, Spencer. "HHS Proposes to Tighten Nursing Home Inspections." *Washington Post*, Section A. 16 November 1987, p. 11.

Rich, Spencer. "Congress Passes Catastrophic Illness Bill." *Washington Post*, Section A. 28 October 1987, p. 1.

Rich, Spencer. "Provisions of 'Catastrophic Insurance Act.'" *Washington Post*, Section A. 1 July 1988, p. 21.

Richardson, Karalee, R.N. "Hope and Flexibility." *Nursing 82*. June 1982, pp. 65–69.

Rivlin, Alice M., and Joshua M. Wiener with Raymond J. Hanley and Denise A. Spence. *Caring for the Disabled Elderly: Who Will Pay?* Washington, D.C.: The Brookings Institution, 1988.

Roettinger, Ruth L. "Living Wills: Real Choice." *Washington Post*, Health Section. 5 April 1988, p. 4.

Seigal, Frederick P., M.D., and Marta Seigal, M.A. *AIDS: The Medical Mystery*. 1st ed. New York: Grove Press, 1983.

Sirrocco, A. Nursing Home Characteristics: 1986 Inventory of Long-Term Care Places. National Center for Health Statistics. Vital Health stat 14(33), 1989.

Siwek, Jay, M.D. "Consultation." *Washington Post*, Health Section. 24 May 1988, p. 21.

Social Security Act. Section 1902 (a)(13)(A).

Stonecypher, D.D., M.D. *Getting Older and Staying Young*. New York: W.W. Norton, 1974.

Stoppard, Miriam, M.D. *The Best Years of Your Life.* 1st ed. New York: Villard Books, 1984.

U.S. Congress. Senate Special Committee on Aging. *Nursing Home Care: The Unfinished Agenda.* 99th Congress, 2nd session. Serial No. 99-J. Washington, D.C.: Government Printing Office, May 1986.

U.S. Department of Health and Human Services. Administration on Aging. "Guidebook for Long-Term Care Ombudsman Reports for FY 1984." 1986.

U.S. Department of Health and Human Services. Administration on Aging. "Long-Term Care Ombudsman Self-Assessment Background Paper. 23 April 1986, p. 3.

U.S. Department of Health and Human Services. Administration on Aging. "National Summary of State Long-Term Care Ombudsman Reports for FY 1984." 11 February 1986.

U.S. Department of Health and Human Services. Health Care Financing Administration. Office of Research and Demonstration. Baltimore, Maryland. Unpublished data, Provider of Service file. 30 December 1989.

U.S. Department of Health and Human Services. Health Care Financing Administration. *Your Medicare Handbook.* Publication #HCFA-10050, ICN-461250. March 1986.

U.S. Department of Health and Human Services. Health Care Financing Administration. *Guide to Health Insurance for People with Medicare.* Publication #02110.

Vladeck, Bruce C. *Unloving Care.* New York: Basic Books, 1980.

Weisberg, Judith, ACSW, LCSW. "A Success Story: Grouping the Alert with the Mentally Impaired." *Geriatric Nursing.* Vol. 5, no. 7. September/October 1984.

Weisberg, Judith, ACSW, LCSW and Maxine R. Haberman, ACSW, LCSW. "Enhancing Self-Esteem of the Young through Grandchildren's Day in a Home for the Aged." *Nursing Homes.* March/April 1987.

Winter, Griffith H., M.D. *Complete Guide to Prescription and Nonprescription Drugs.* Tucson, Ariz.: H.P. Books, 1983.

Index

AARP: *See* American Association of Retired People

Abuse, physical and psychological, 113–117

Acquired Immune Deficiency (AIDS): *See* Medical problems

Administration on Aging, 137

Administrators, 30, 31–33
  handling problems with, 117–120
  responsibilities of, 32
  staff relationship, 32–33
  and talking with while touring facility, 53

Admission, 78–93
  adjustment period concerning, 89–93
  and the first day, 87–89
  information to take upon, 81
  involuntary, 8–9
  paperwork, 83–84
  and personal care notes, 81
  preparations for, 80–83
  what not to bring upon, 86–87
  what to bring upon, 84–85

The AIDS Clearing House, 127

Alternative living situations, 11–12

Alzheimer's disease:
  Medicaid special benefits for, 99
  special programs for, 98–99

Alzheimer's Disease and Related Disorders Association (ADRDA), 65, 99

American Association of Retired Persons (AARP), 65, 84

Arthritis: *See* Medical problems

Bill of Rights, resident's, 138–139
  and example of complaint procedure, 140

Cancer: *See* Medical problems

Care:
  evaluating quality of, 54–60
  inadequate, 113–117
  and interdisciplinary patient care plan, 46–47
  personal, 81
  see also Medical care and treatment

Certified medicine aides (CMA), 37, 56
  responsibilities of, 38

Charge nurses: *See* Clinical nurse managers

Clinical nurse managers, 36–37
  handling problems with, 118–119
  responsibilities of, 37
  and talking with while touring facility, 54

Department of Health and Human Services (DHHS), 25

Dietitians, 43–44
  responsibilities of, 44

Director of Nurses, 30, 34–36
  handling problems with, 118
  responsibilities of, 36

Disability: *See* Disease and disability

Discharges, 109–111
  handling of, 110–111
  reasons for, 109–110
  without physician's order, 110

Disease and disability:
  questions and answers concerning, 98–103

Division of Elder Affairs, 109

Doctors: *See* Physicians

Drugs: *See* Medications

Dying, 125–134
  five stages of, 128–133
  and when death occurs, 133–
    134

Elderly:
  factors warranting nursing home
    care for, 6–10
  and feelings about moving into
    nursing home, 78–80
  statistics concerning, 5–6
  see also Residents, nursing
    home

Financing the care, 63–77
  and average cost of nursing
    home care, 65–67
  changes in, 65
  fraudulent charges concerning,
    75–77
  and Medicaid, 63, 72–75
  and Medicare, 63, 67–72
  and questions to ask of a
    nursing home, 61–62
  using private sources, 65–67
  and Veterans Administration
    funding, 64

Group living, 9

Handicapped: See Disease and
    disability
Head nurses: See Clinical nurse
    managers
Health care: See Care; Medical
    care and treatment
Health Care and Financing
    Administration (HCFA), 26, 67,
    72, 73, 83
Health facility licensing and
    certification directors, directory
    of, 149–159

"Improving the Quality of Care in
    Nursing Homes" (report), 135–
    136
Inadequate care: See Abuse,
    physical and psychological
Inspections, government, 19–25
  of employment practices, 24
  examples of questions asked by
    inspectors during, 21
  examples of what checked
    during, 24

reports, 25–26
  of residents rights, 22–24
Institute of Medicine (IoM), 3
Interdisciplinary patient care plan,
    46–47

Kübler-Ross, Elizabeth, 125, 128

"Long-Term Care Survey Process"
    (LTCSP), 25–26

Medicaid, 63, 72–75
  impoverishment protection, 73
  and special benefits for
    Alzheimer's disease, 99
  see also Medicare
Medical care and treatment:
  information to take upon
    admission concerning, 81
  residents rights concerning, 22–
    23
  supplemental services
    concerning, 105–107
Medical directors, 30, 33–34
Medical problems:
  AIDS, 125, 126–127
  alcoholism, 102
  Alzheimer's disease, 98–99
  arthritis, 103
  blindness, 102–103
  cancer, 103–105
  constipation, 97
  edema, 96
  flu, 95–96
  heart disease, 101–102
  infections, 95–96
  injuries, 100
  mental illness, 9
  Parkinson's disease, 100–101
  pneumonia, 95
  pressure sores, 97
  prostatitis, 95
  shingles, 95–96
  strokes, 101–102
  urinary tract infections, 96
  vaginitis, 95
  weight loss, 94
Medicare, 63, 67–72
  denial letter, sample, 69
  hotline number, 72
  information sources, 72
  Part A, 68–71
  Part B, 71–72
  services covered by Part A, 71

services covered by Part B, 71
services not covered by Part A, 70
services not covered by Part B, 72
supplemental coverage, 72
and taking resident out of facility, 71
who is eligible for, 67
see also Medicaid
"Medicare Supplement Insurance Guide," 72
Medications, 86, 164–167
commonly used in geriatrics (table), 165–166
and having personal pharmacist filling prescriptions, 105–106
medical "cocktail," 104
for pain control, 103–105
"Medigap" plans, 72

National Association of Boards of Nursing Home Examiners, 32
National Citizens' Coalition for Nursing Home Reform (NCCNHR), 65, 123, 136, 137
National Council on Aging, 12
National Institute of Aging, 12, 125
Neglect: *See* Abuse, physical and psychological
Nursing assistants, 38–39
handling problems with, 119
responsibilities of, 38
Nursing Home Reform Law, 16
Nursing homes:
admission, 78–93
average cost of care in, 65–67
choosing, 48–62
chronic care, 17–18
and citizen involvement for reforming, 136–137
comparing, 60–62
decision to look for, 5–10
discharge from, 109–111
dying in, 125–134
employment practices, 24
evaluating quality of care in, 55–60
financial questions to ask of, 61
and government action for reforming, 135–136
handling of problems with, 112–124

inspections of, 19–25
and interdisciplinary patient care plan, 46–47
intermediate care, 16, 17
location, 62
multilevel, 17
nonproprietary, 18
personal care, 16
proprietary, 18
skilled care, 16, 17
staff, 30–47
substandard, 26–29
that are not licensed and certified, 18–19
touring, 50–60
transferring, 107–108
types of, 15–19
see also Services offered
Nursing staff: *See* Staff, nursing home

Older Women's League, 65
On Death and Dying (Kübler-Ross), 125, 128
Orderlies: *See* Nursing assistants
Organ donations, 82

Pain control:
for arthritis, 103
for cancer, 103–105
medical "cocktail," 104
for nonresponsive residents, 105
patient-controlled analgesia, 104–105
Parkinson's disease: *See* Medical problems
Patients: *See* Residents, nursing home
Personal Care:
information to take upon admission, 81
Personal funds:
residents rights concerning, 24–25
Personal items, 85–86
Physicians:
handling problems with, 120–121
Privacy:
residents rights concerning, 22–23
Problems, handling, 112–124
of abuse, 113–117

with physicians, 120–121
and questions to ask before
    leaving a nursing home, 124
with staff members, 117–120
of theft, 115–116
and what to do, 121–124

Quality assurance program, 23–24
Quality of life, 1–5
    measuring, 3

Referrals, nursing home:
    sources of, 49–50
Residents, nursing home:
    Bill of Rights, 138–139
    care and treatment; rights
        concerning, 22–23
    disoriented, 56–57
    nonresponsive; pain control for,
        105
    personal funds; rights
        concerning, 24–25
    privacy; rights concerning, 22–
        23
    sexuality; rights concerning, 22–
        23
    staff interaction, 55–56
    and talking with while touring
        facility, 53
    see also Elderly
Resource centers, 160–163
Room and board, 16
Rooms, residents', 52
    changing, 109

"Self-Care and Self-Help Groups
    for the Elderly: A Directory,"
    12
Services offered:
    activities, 57–59
    barber shops, 53
    beauty shops, 53
    dental, 107
    housekeeping, 45
    laboratory, 107
    laundry, 45
    maintenance, 45, 50
    meals, 57
    medical, 22, 81, 105–107

podiatry, 106–107
spas, 53
x-ray, 107
Sexuality:
    residents rights concerning, 22–
        23
Shingles (herpes zoster): See
    Medical problems
Social Security Administration, 67
Social workers, 39–40
    responsibilities of, 40
    and talking with when choosing
        a facility, 53–54
Staff, nursing home, 30–47
    activities director, 40–41
    administrator, 30, 31–33
    attire of, 54
    certified medicine aide, 37
    clinical nurse manager, 36–37
    dietitian, 43–44
    director of nurses, 30, 34–36
    handling problems with, 117–
        124
    housekeepers, 45
    laundry workers, 45
    maintenance workers, 45
    medical director, 30, 33–34
    nursing assistant, 38–39
    resident interaction, 55–56
    social worker, 39–40
    and talking with while touring
        facility, 53–54
    therapists, 42–43
State agencies on aging, directory
    of, 141–148
Strokes: See Medical problems

Therapists, 42–43
    occupational, 42–43
    physical, 42, 43
    speech, 42, 43

U.S. Senate Special Committee on
    Aging, 4, 25, 99
    on substandard nursing homes,
        26–29

Veterans Administration funding,
    64